COVID-19 Drug Development - Recent Advances, New Perspectives and Applications

Edited by Arli Aditya Parikesit

Published in London, United Kingdom

COVID-19 Drug Development - Recent Advances, New Perspectives and Applications
http://dx.doi.org/10.5772/intechopen.100969
Edited by Arli Aditya Parikesit

Contributors
Vivek Puri, Ameya Sharma, Sandeep Puri, Varun Puri, Divya Dheer, Neha Bhandari, Nicolás Padilla-Raygoza, Maria De Jesus Gallardo-Luna, Efrain Navarro-Olivos, Francisco Javier Magos-Vazquez, Daniel Alberto Diaz-Martinez, Gilberto Flores-Vargas, Jalpa Suthar, Jhanvi Patel, Shubham Atal, Ananyan Sampath, Aditya Banerjee, Ratinder Jhaj, Matias Nunes Frizzo, Thiago Gomes Heck, Mirna Stela Stela Ludwig, Pauline Brendler Goettems Fiorin, Joise Wottrich, Eduardo Gonçalves, Carina Echer De Souza, Arli Aditya Parikesit, Rizky Nurdiansyah, Amornrat Ratanasiri, Pissamai Homchampa, Khemika Napattaradechanon, Parichat Yatniyom, Thawalrat Ratanasiri, Piyaporn Sansila, Thanawan Sirisuk, Thawalwong Ratanasiri, Kenneth Bitrus David, Yusuff Olnarewaju Azeez, Cynthia Chidera Okafor

First published in London, United Kingdom, 2022 by IntechOpen
IntechOpen is the global imprint of INTECHOPEN LIMITED, registered in England and Wales, registration number: 11086078, 5 Princes Gate Court, London, SW7 2QJ, United Kingdom

British Library Cataloguing-in-Publication Data
A catalogue record for this book is available from the British Library

Additional hard and PDF copies can be obtained from orders@intechopen.com

COVID-19 Drug Development - Recent Advances, New Perspectives and Applications
Edited by Arli Aditya Parikesit
p. cm.
Print ISBN 978-1-80356-989-5
Online ISBN 978-1-80356-990-1
eBook (PDF) ISBN 978-1-80356-991-8

Meet the editor

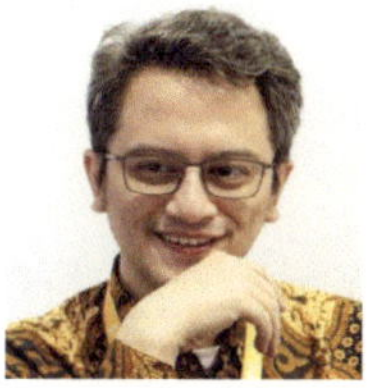

Arli Aditya Parikesit is the Vice-Rector of Research and Innovation at the Indonesia International Institute for Life Sciences (I3L). He received his bachelor's and master's degrees in chemistry from the Faculty of Mathematics and Natural Sciences, University of Indonesia. His doctoral research at the Bioinformatics Group, Faculty of Informatics and Mathematics, University of Leipzig, Germany is focused on the utilization of modern protein domain annotation techniques for the three domains of life. Dr. Arli is also an expert on immunoinformatics, bioinformatics algorithms, structural bioinformatics, in-silico drug design, and in-silico transcriptomics. Currently, Dr. Arli is applying his expertise to the development of a COVID-19 drug and vaccine design pipeline.

Contents

Preface

As of 27 September 2022, there have been more than 612 million confirmed cases of COVID-19, including more than 6.5 million deaths reported to WHO. Although complete sets of diagnostics, drugs, and vaccines are already in place, public health systems in many parts of the world are currently still under strain due to the effect of the pandemic. Moreover, many countries and territories are already advising the reopening of their economies, and the relaxation of health protocols including mask-wearing and social distancing. Scientists already predict that COVID-19 will move into an endemic phase, although not in the near future. The SARS-CoV-2 virus is not likely to be eradicated during our lifetime. As has been seen with influenza viruses, such as H1N1, the re-emergence of this virus into a future epidemic is possible. Therefore, research to design novel therapies for COVID-19 remains necessary, as the mutational trajectory of SARS-CoV-2 is difficult to predict. New variants may well emerge in the future, and any drug development program should always be aligned accordingly.

This book seeks to make an intellectual contribution to this ongoing pandemic. It is divided into three sections. First, the introductory section elaborates on the importance of drug development for COVID-19. Second, specific unique cases in clinical settings are reported. The final section, on case treatment and management, takes a more comprehensive health sciences approach. Some of the contributions cover extensive ongoing research and development that will encourage further debate on the management of the COVID-19 pandemic.

I would like to express my gratitude to Rizky Nurdiansyah, MSi, Head of Research and Community Service Development at the Indonesia International Institute for Life Sciences, for interesting discussions and excellent collaboration in the field of COVID-19 drug design. Thanks also go to the students of the School of Life Sciences, Indonesia International Institute for Life Sciences, for their heartfelt motivation.

Arli Aditya Parikesit
Department of Bioinformatics,
School of Life Sciences,
Indonesia International Institute for Life Sciences,
Jakarta, Indonesia

Section 1

Introduction

Chapter 1

Introductory Chapter: Current Perspective of COVID-19 Drugs

Arli Aditya Parikesit and Rizky Nurdiansyah

1. Introduction

1.1 Early efforts of drug repurposing

When WHO declared that the COVID-19 pandemic was in place on March 2020, there were no standard drugs available for this new disease. One of the fastest and the most effective solution to face this problem is relying on the drug repurposing effort. Remdesivir is one of the earliest repurposed drug, as it has been originally develop for hepatitis C, and already examined for application in Ebola and Marburg virus infection [1, 2]. In the laboratory setting, remdesivir has been proven to inhibit the RdRp protein of SARS-CoV-2 that is responsible for viral replication, shortens hospitalization period, and is supported with vivid computational model [2–5]. Hence, remdesivir could only be provided in hospital as it should be delivered intravenously to the patients, thus deterring out-patient application [6]. In parallel, some other repurposing efforts are on the way as well.

These anti-worm and anti-parasitic drugs, Ivermectin, Chloroquine, and Hydroxychloroquine, are also repurposed. Although they provide promising in vitro and in vivo leads, there are inconclusive clinical trial results. Moreover, some meta-analysis results provide some leads that are yet to be validated in the clinical trials [7–12]. Hence, there are some repurposed drugs that are efficacious to reduce the severe effects of COVID-19, although they are not anti-viral ones. Dexamethasone, a long-standing standard drug of anti-inflammation and anti-coagulation, could inhibit the 'cytokine storm' of late stage COVID-19 [13]. It also acts as immune modulator as well [14, 15]. Then, Heparin that works as anti-blot clot drug, also deployed to the COVID-19 patients [16–19]. However, during the early phase of COVID-19 pandemics, there are no standard drugs that could provide solid clinical evidence and could be deployed in out-patients.

2. Ascendancy of standard drugs for COVID-19

The development of Paxlovid and Molnupiravir, both of them are synthetic drugs, have enabled new standard due to the emergency FDA's authorization [20, 21]. As nucleoside analogue, molnupiravir has successfully inhibited RdRp protein of SARS-CoV-2 while providing significant clinical trials result for patients with mild-to-moderate symptoms of COVID-19 [22]. Thus, Paxlovid, which is a combination of two distinctive drugs of nirmatrelvir dan ritonavir, could inhibit SARS-CoV-2's main protease enzyme with retaining its acceptable concentration in the blood, and reduces hospital admission alongside with mortality rate significantly [23, 24]. Hence, both drugs were optimized with rational drug design methods and approved by the FDA with emergency authorization [22–26]. Although remdesivir has provided significant efficacy in the clinical setting, its in-patient setting prevented the wide-spread use. However, the development of oral remdesivir has been devised and the current status is deemed successful in the in vivo trials [27, 28]. Although careful and thorough examination by medical specialist is necessary before deploying those anti-viral drugs, they are considered the available standard drugs for COVID-19 so far.

3. FAERS database annotation of COVID-19 drug trials

FDA Adverse Event Reporting System (FAERS) Public Dashboard is the Bioinformatics approach in curating side effects of drug trials from clinical data [29, 30]. It has special public dashboard for COVID-19 emergency use authorization (EUA) products, as seen in the **Figure 1**.

The FAERS database has annotated COVID-19 drug trials side effects, such as the trials with hydroxychloroquine/chloroquine, bamlanivimab, Ribavirin-Interferon and ivermectin [31–37]. Moreover, cancer patients who were old (65 year-old and above), males, and taking immunosuppressive treatment, as well as those with hematological malignancies, were at a higher risk of death due to COVID-19 infection, according to FAERS data [34]. Hence, pertaining the existing COVID-19 standard drugs, the finding in FAERS database did not affect current FDA's endorsement as it is considered still a relatively novel development. More trials will be necessary. Thus, extensive computational and wet lab studies of the leads' pharmacological and toxicological properties should be carefully examined [38].

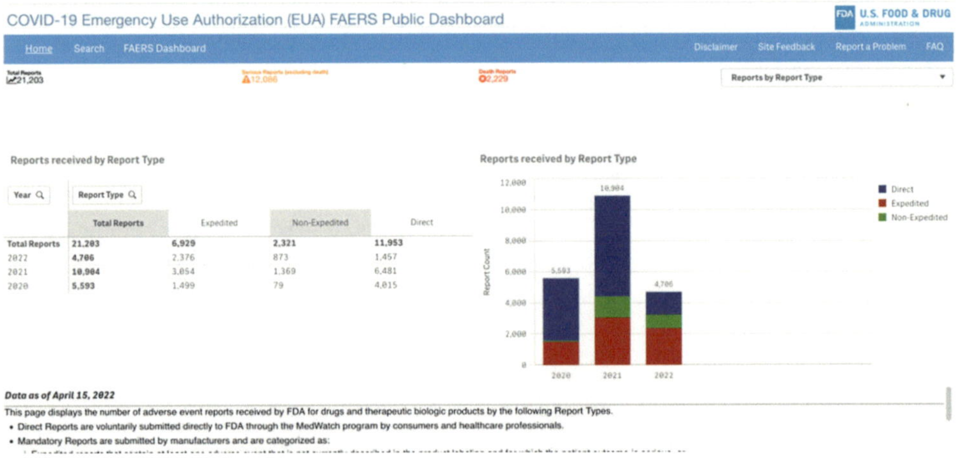

Figure 1.
COVID-19 emergency use authorization (EUA) FAERS public dashboard (source: https://www.fda.gov/drugs/questions-and-answers-fdas-adverse-event-reporting-system-faers/fda-adverse-event-reporting-system-faers-public-dashboard).

4. Promise of natural product leads

Since the early phase of the pandemics, many researchers have tried to examine bioactive compounds such as propolis and others, from natural products source as leads for SARS-CoV-2 drug candidates [39–47]. Although these efforts are still on going up to now, the leads are still in experimental stage in general. Several leads were developed with computational approaches from natural products, albeit still no conclusive experimental evidence that leads into clinical trials [48–51]. There is also effort for repurposing natural product leads, from H5N1 inhibitor lead compounds, that are yet to provide wet lab results [52]. One example of the lead compound with in silico potential for inhibiting SARS-CoV-2 is Juglanin, as visualized in **Figure 2**.

Computation of natural products chemistry is a way to leverage the indigenous knowledge with modern science such as bioinformatics and biomedicine [48, 54–63]. It has achieve certain success in medical application, such as the chemotherapy agent of Taxol [64, 65]. However, there is no standard natural product-based drug yet for COVID-19 up to now. In general, existing COVID-19 standard drugs are repurposed drugs that mainly comprises of synthetic and semi-synthetic compounds [66, 67]. How natural products bioactive compounds will perform in this domain, it remains to be seen.

5. Coronavirus and anticipation of future pandemics

The SARS, MERS, and COVID-19 pandemics have taught us valuable lessons that coronavirus outbreak could not be underestimated. This particular virus has showcased themselves as constant menace to the public health. Therefore, it would need

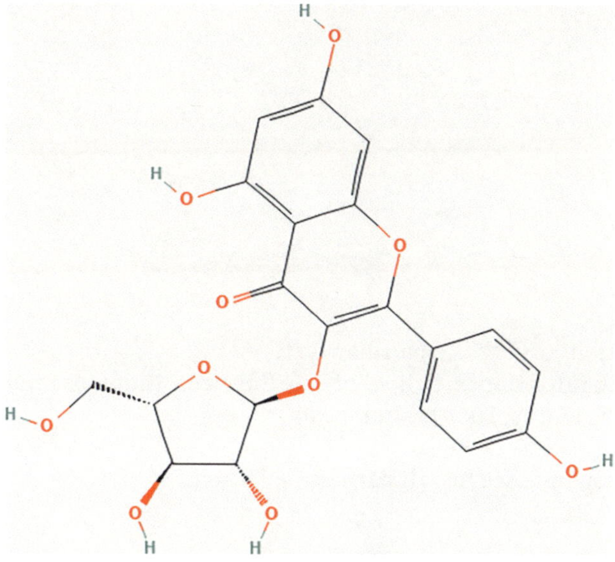

Figure 2.
Juglanin, provided as the lead for SARS-CoV-2 drug candidate based on in silico approach [53] (source: https://pubchem.ncbi.nlm.nih.gov/compound/5318717#section=2D-Structure).

establishment of a dedicated research network world-wide to cater this challenge. The current pandemics has been predicted in quite a while. Based on WHO guidelines in 2015, it is stated explicitly that coronavirus has a prospect of becoming pandemic [68, 69]. There are hundreds or even thousands coronavirus species that potentially some of them could be spilled to human population from animals [68, 69]. Although conclusive evidence is still gathered on the moment, the existing leads are pointing to the spill over of coronavirus from bat as precursor of this on-going pandemic [70–73]. As a RNA virus, it has high mutation rate for the genetic material, and as new SARS-CoV-2 variants emerged, it elicits potential to tamper the efficacy of the existing therapy [74–77]. In these uncertain conditions, Biologics and/or biosimilars such as monoclonal antibody, polypeptide, and protein-based therapy are proposed as potential therapies for COVID-19 infections. Their high bioavailability in the cell is one of the strength in the pharmacokinetics properties [78]. Monoclonal antibodies therapy has been proven to provide good efficacy against COVID-19 in clinical setting [79, 80]. Moreover, some peptide-based leads are currently under development as COVID-19 drug candidates [81]. For siRNA, some in silico and wet lab research are underway, albeit the clinical application is yet to be determined [82–84]. In this end, more variative approaches are available as means to anticipate future coronavirus pandemics.

Acknowledgements

The authors would like to express their gratitude to the Indonesia International Institute for Life Sciences (i3L) Department of Research and Community Service (LPPM) for their support of this study. The authors wish to express their gratitude to the Direktorat Sumber Daya, Kementerian Pendidikan, Kebudayaan, dan Ristek, as well as LLDIKTI3, for giving Hibah Penelitian Dasar Berbasis Kompetensi 2022 No. 0054/E5/AK.04/2022.

Author details

Arli Aditya Parikesit* and Rizky Nurdiansyah
Department of Bioinformatics, School of Life Sciences, Indonesia International Institute for Life Sciences, Jakarta, Indonesia

*Address all correspondence to: arli.parikesit@i3l.ac.id

References

[1] Malin JJ, Suárez I, Priesner V, Fätkenheuer G, Rybniker J. Remdesivir against COVID-19 and other viral diseases. Clinical Microbiology Reviews. 2021;**34**(1):1-21. DOI: 10.1128/CMR.00162-20

[2] Eastman RT et al. Remdesivir: A review of its discovery and development leading to emergency use authorization for treatment of COVID-19. ACS Central Science. 2020;**6**(5):672. DOI: 10.1021/ACSCENTSCI.0C00489

[3] Parikesit AA, Nurdiansyah R. Drug repurposing option for COVID-19 with structural bioinformatics of chemical interactions approach. Cermin Dunia Kedokteran. 2020;**47**(3):222-226. DOI: 10.5281/zenodo.4460736

[4] Shannon A et al. Remdesivir and SARS-CoV-2: Structural requirements at both nsp12 RdRp and nsp14 exonuclease active-sites. Antiviral Research. 2020;**178**:104793. DOI: 10.1016/j.antiviral.2020.104793

[5] Arba M, Wahyudi ST, Brunt DJ, Paradis N, Wu C. Mechanistic insight on the remdesivir binding to RNA-dependent RNA polymerase (RdRp) of SARS-cov-2. Computers in Biology and Medicine. 2021;**129**:104156. DOI: 10.1016/j.compbiomed.2020.104156

[6] Gottlieb RL et al. Early Remdesivir to prevent progression to severe Covid-19 in outpatients. New England Journal of Medicine. 2021;**386**(4):305-315. DOI: 10.1056/NEJMOA2116846

[7] Chosidow O et al. Ivermectin as a potential treatment for COVID-19? PLoS Neglected Tropical Diseases. 2021;**15**(6):e0009446. DOI: 10.1371/journal.pntd.0009446

[8] Food and Drug Administration (FDA). Why You Should Not Use Ivermectin to Treat or Prevent COVID-19. Coronavirus. 2021. Available from: https://www.fda.gov/consumers/consumer-updates/why-you-should-not-use-ivermectin-treat-or-prevent-covid-19 [Accessed: June 10, 2021]

[9] WHO. WHO Advises that Ivermectin only be used to Treat COVID-19 Within Clinical Trials. Feature stories. 2021. Available from: https://www.who.int/news-room/feature-stories/detail/who-advises-that-ivermectin-only-be-used-to-treat-covid-19-within-clinical-trials [Accessed: June 10, 2021]

[10] Meyerowitz-Katz G, Wieten S, Arellano M d JM, Yamey G. Unethical studies of ivermectin for covid-19. BMJ. 2022;**377**:o917. DOI: 10.1136/bmj.o917

[11] Ahmed S et al. A five-day course of ivermectin for the treatment of COVID-19 may reduce the duration of illness. International Journal of Infectious Diseases. 2021;**103**:214-216. DOI: 10.1016/j.ijid.2020.11.191

[12] Caly L, Druce JD, Catton MG, Jans DA, Wagstaff KM. The FDA-approved drug ivermectin inhibits the replication of SARS-CoV-2 in vitro. Antiviral Research. 2020;**178**:104787. DOI: 10.1016/j.antiviral.2020.104787

[13] Sharun K, Tiwari R, Dhama J, Dhama K. Dexamethasone to combat cytokine storm in COVID-19: Clinical trials and preliminary evidence. International Journal of Surgery (London, England). 2020;**82**:179. DOI: 10.1016/J.IJSU.2020.08.038

[14] WHO. Coronavirus Disease (COVID-19): Dexamethasone. Geneva:

World Health Organization; 2020. Available from: https://www.who.int/news-room/q-a-detail/coronavirus-disease-covid-19-dexamethasone [Accessed: July 13, 2021]

[15] Ahmed MH, Hassan A. Dexamethasone for the treatment of coronavirus disease (COVID-19): A review. SN Comprehensive Clinical Medicine. 2020;**2**(12):2637-2646. DOI: 10.1007/s42399-020-00610-8

[16] Hippensteel JA, LaRiviere WB, Colbert JF, Langou t-Astri CJ, Schmidt EP. Heparin as a therapy for COVID-19: Current evidence and future possibilities. American Journal of Physiology - Lung Cellular and Molecular Physiology. 2020;**319**(2):L211. DOI: 10.1152/AJPLUNG.00199.2020

[17] Billett HH et al. Anticoagulation in COVID-19: Effect of enoxaparin, heparin, and Apixaban on mortality. Thrombosis and Haemostasis. 2020;**120**(12):1691. DOI: 10.1055/S-0040-1720978

[18] Garcia Azorin D.Guidance for clinical case management of thrombosis with thrombocytopenia syndrome (TTS) following vaccination to prevent coronavirus disease (COVID-19). WHO COVID-19 Task Force. 2021

[19] ten Cate H. Surviving Covid-19 with heparin? New England Journal of Medicine. 2021;**385**(9):845-846. DOI: 10.1056/NEJME2111151/SUPPL_FILE/NEJME2111151_DISCLOSURES.PDF

[20] FDA COVID-19 Task Force. Coronavirus (COVID-19) Update: FDA Authorizes First Oral Antiviral for Treatment of COVID-19. Maryland, US: FDA; 2022. Available from: https://www.fda.gov/news-events/press-announcements/coronavirus-covid-19-update-fda-authorizes-first-oral-antiviral-treatment-covid-19; [Accessed: April 21, 2022]

[21] FDA COVID-19 Task Force. Coronavirus (COVID-19) Update: FDA Authorizes Additional Oral Antiviral for Treatment of COVID-19 in Certain Adults. Maryland, US: FDA; 2022. Available from: https://www.fda.gov/news-events/press-announcements/coronavirus-covid-19-update-fda-authorizes-additional-oral-antiviral-treatment-covid-19-certain; [Accessed: April 21, 2022]

[22] Masyeni S et al. Molnupiravir: A lethal mutagenic drug against rapidly mutating SARS-CoV-2 – A narrative review. Journal of Medical Virology. 2022;**94**(7):3006-3016. DOI: 10.1002/jmv.27730

[23] Wang Z, Yang L. In the age of omicron variant: Paxlovid raises new hopes of COVID-19 recovery. Journal of Medical Virology. 2021;**94**(5):1766-1767. DOI: 10.1002/JMV.27540

[24] Mahase E. Covid-19: Pfizer's paxlovid is 89% effective in patients at risk of serious illness, company reports. BMJ. 2021;**375**:n2713. DOI: 10.1136/BMJ.N2713

[25] Cave JA, Phizackerley D. Molnupiravir: Evidence by press release. Drug and Therapeutics Bulletin. 2022;**60**(1):2-2. DOI: 10.1136/DTB.2021.000064

[26] Fischer W et al. Molnupiravir, an Oral antiviral treatment for COVID-19. medRxiv. 2021;**1**:1-5. DOI: 10.1101/2021.06.17.21258639

[27] Schäfer A et al. Therapeutic treatment with an oral prodrug of the remdesivir parental nucleoside is protective against SARS-CoV-2

pathogenesis in mice. Science Translational Medicine. 2022;**14**(643):1-5 DOI: 10.1126/scitranslmed.abm3410

[28] Cox RM et al. Oral prodrug of remdesivir parent GS-441524 is efficacious against SARS-CoV-2 in ferrets. Nature Communications. 2021;**12**(1):1-11. DOI: 10.1038/s41467-021-26760-4

[29] FDA COVID-19 Task Force. FDA Launches FAERS Dashboard for COVID-19 Therapies. Maryland, US: RAPS; 2022. Available from: https://www.raps.org/ news-and-articles/news-articles/2021/3/fda-launches-faers-dashboard-for-covid-19-therapie; [Accessed: March 17, 2022]

[30] Veronin MA, Schumaker RP, Dixit R. The irony of MedWatch and the FAERS database: An assessment of data input errors and potential consequences. Journal of Pharmacy Technology. (SAGE Publications Sage CA: Los Angeles, CA) 2020;**36**(4) 164-167. DOI: 10.1177/8755122520928495

[31] Yuan J et al. Pharmacotherapy management for COVID-19 and cardiac safety: A data mining approach for pharmacovigilance evidence from the FDA adverse event reporting system (FAERS). Drugs - Real World Outcomes. 2021;**8**(2):131-140. DOI: 10.1007/s40801-021-00229-8

[32] Shan W, Hong D, Zhu J, Zhao Q. Assessment of the potential adverse events related to ribavirin-interferon combination for novel coronavirus therapy. Computational and Mathematical Methods in Medicine. 2020;**2020**:1-7. DOI: 10.1155/2020/1391583

[33] Guo W et al. Informing selection of drugs for COVID-19 treatment through adverse events analysis. Scientific Reports. 2021;**11**(1):1-7. DOI: 10.1038/s41598-021-93500-5

[34] Abdel-Rahman O. Factors associated with fatal coronavirus disease 2019 infections among cancer patients in the US FDA adverse event reporting system database. Future Oncology. 2021;**17**(36):5045-5051. DOI: 10.2217/fon-2021-0816

[35] Zhao Y et al. Serious cardiovascular adverse events associated with hydroxychloroquine/chloroquine alone or with azithromycin in patients with COVID-19: A pharmacovigilance analysis of the FDA adverse event reporting system (FAERS). Drugs - Real World Outcomes. 2022;**2022**:1-11. DOI: 10.1007/S40801-022-00300-Y

[36] Tuccori M et al. An overview of the preclinical discovery and development of bamlanivimab for the treatment of novel coronavirus infection (COVID-19): Reasons for limited clinical use and lessons for the future. Expert Opinion on Drug Discovery. 2021;**16**(12):1403-1414. DOI: 10.1080/17460441.2021.1960819

[37] Perez J, Roustit M, Lepelley M, Revol B, Cracowski JL, Khouri C. Reported adverse drug reactions associated with the use of hydroxychloroquine and chloroquine during the COVID-19 pandemic. Annals of Internal Medicine. 2021;**174**(6):878-880. DOI: 10.7326/M20-7918

[38] Geerts T, vander Heyden Y. In silico predictions of ADME-Tox properties: Drug absorption. Combinatorial Chemistry & High Throughput Screening. 2011;**14**(5):339-361

[39] Bachevski D, Damevska K, Simeonovski V, Dimova M. Back to the basics: Propolis and COVID-19. Dermatologic Therapy. 2020;**33**(4):100-115. DOI: 10.1111/dth.13780

[40] Berretta AA, Silveira MAD, Cóndor Capcha JM, de Jong D. Propolis and its potential against SARS-CoV-2 infection mechanisms and COVID-19 disease: Running title: Propolis against SARS-CoV-2 infection and COVID-19. Biomedicine and Pharmacotherapy. (Elsevier Masson SAS) 2020;**131**:110622. DOI: 10.1016/j.biopha.2020.110622

[41] Sahlan M, al Faris MNH, Aditama R, Lischer K, Khayrani AC, Pratami DK. Molecular docking of South Sulawesi Propolis against fructose 1,6-Bisphosphatase as a type 2 diabetes mellitus drug. International Journal of Technology. 2020;**11**(5):910. DOI: 10.14716/ijtech.v11i5.4332

[42] Güler HI, Tatar G, Yildiz O, Belduz AO. An investigation of ethanolic propolis extracts: Their potential inhibitor properties against ACE-II receptors for COVID-19 treatment by molecular docking study. ScienceOpen. 2020;**1**:1-5

[43] Arba M et al. Virtual screening of the Indonesian medicinal plant and zinc databases for potential inhibitors of the RNA-dependent RNA polymerase (RdRp) of 2019 novel coronavirus. Indonesian Journal of Chemistry. 2020;**20**(6):1430. DOI: 10.22146/ijc.56120

[44] Shivanika C, Kumar D, Ragunathan V, Tiwari P, Sumitha A, Devi B. Molecular docking, validation, dynamics simulations, and pharmacokinetic prediction of natural compounds against the SARS-CoV-2 main-protease. Journal of Biomolecular Structure and Dynamics. 2020;**40**(2):585-611. DOI: 10.1080/07391102.2020.1815584

[45] Sukardiman M, Ervina MF, Pratama HP, Siswodihardjo S. The coronavirus disease 2019 main protease inhibitor from Andrographis paniculata (Burm.f) ness. Journal of Advanced Pharmaceutical Technology & Research. 2020;**11**(4):157. DOI: 10.4103/japtr.japtr_84_20

[46] Zhang D, Wu K, Zhang X, Deng S, Peng B. In silico screening of Chinese herbal medicines with the potential to directly inhibit 2019 novel coronavirus. Journal of Integrative Medicine. 2020;**18**(2):152-158. DOI: 10.1016/j.joim.2020.02.005

[47] Pang W et al. Chinese medical drugs for coronavirus disease 2019: A systematic review and meta-analysis. Integrative Medicine Research. 2020;**9**(3):100477. DOI: 10.1016/j.imr.2020.100477

[48] Wijaya R, Hafidzhah M, Kharisma V, Ansori A, Parikesit A. COVID-19 In silico drug with Zingiber officinale natural product compound library targeting the Mpro protein. Makara Journal of Science. 2021;**25**(3):5. DOI: 10.7454/mss.v25i3.1244

[49] Dibha AF et al. Biological activity of kencur (Kaempferia galanga L.) against SARS-CoV-2 main protease. International Journal of Health Sciences. 2022;**6**(S1):468-480. DOI: 10.53730/IJHS.V6NS1.4779

[50] Ansori A et al. Bioactive compounds from Mangosteen (Garcinia mangostana L.) as an antiviral agent via dual inhibitor mechanism against SARSCoV- 2: An In silico approach. Pharmacognosy Journal. 2022;**14**(1):85-90. DOI: 10.5530/pj.2022.14.12

[51] Shiloputra AF, Parikesit AA, Darmawan JT, Pricillia V, Turista DDR, Ansori ANM. An overview of the curcumin-based and Allicin bioactive compounds as potential treatment to SARS-CoV-2 with structural

bioinformatics tools. Jurnal Teknologi Laboratorium. 2021;**10**(2):95-101. DOI: 10.29238/TEKNOLABJOURNAL.V10I2.291

[52] Parikesit AA, Nurdiansyah R. Natural products repurposing of the H5N1-based lead compounds for the most fit inhibitors against 3C-like protease of SARS-CoV-2. Journal of Pharmacy & Pharmacognosy Research. 2021;**9**(5):730-745. DOI: 10.5281/zenodo.5529215

[53] Adisurja GP, Parkesit AA. Virtual screening of the flavonoids compounds with the SARS-CoV-2 3C-like protease as the Lead compounds for the COVID-19. Coronaviruses. 2021;**02**(11):1-9. DOI: 10.2174/26 66796702666210222105547

[54] Fadli A, Kusuma WA, Annisa IB, Heryanto R. Screening of potential Indonesia herbal compounds based on multi-label classification for 2019 coronavirus disease. Big Data and Cognitive Computing. 2021;**5**(4):75. DOI: 10.3390/bdcc5040075

[55] Yu MJ. Natural product-like virtual libraries: Recursive atom-based enumeration. Journal of Chemical Information and Modeling. 2011;**51**(3):541-557. DOI: 10.1021/ci1002087

[56] Bauer RA, Wurst JM, Tan DS. Expanding the range of 'druggable' targets with natural product-based libraries: An academic perspective. Current Opinion in Chemical Biology. 2010;**14**(3):308-314. DOI: 10.1016/j.cbpa.2010.02.001

[57] Arakawa T, Yamasaki H, Ikeda K, Ejima D, Naito T, Koyama AH. Antiviral and virucidal activities of natural products. Current Medicinal Chemistry. 2009;**16**(20):2485-2497

[58] Chemat F, Vian MA, Cravotto G. Green extraction of natural products: Concept and principles. International Journal of Molecular Sciences. 2012;**13**(7):8615-8627. DOI: 10.3390/ijms13078615

[59] Cragg GM, Newman DJ. Natural products: A continuing source of novel drug leads. Biochimica et Biophysica Acta. 2013;**1830**(6):3670-3695. DOI: 10.1016/j.bbagen.2013.02.008

[60] Mishra BB, Tiwari VK. Natural products: An evolving role in future drug discovery. European Journal of Medicinal Chemistry. 2011;**46**(10):4769-4807. DOI: 10.1016/j.ejmech.2011.07.057

[61] Zhao H, Medema MH. Standardization for natural product synthetic biology. Natural Product Reports. 2016;**33**(8):920-924. DOI: 10.1039/C6NP00030D

[62] Medema MH, Fischbach MA. Computational approaches to natural product discovery. Nature Chemical Biology. 2015;**11**(9):639-648. DOI: 10.1038/nchembio.1884

[63] Amit Koparde A, Chandrashekar Doijad R, Shripal Magdum C. Natural products in drug discovery. In: Pharmacognosy - Medicinal Plants. London, UK: IntechOpen; 2019. DOI: 10.5772/intechopen.82860

[64] Expósito O et al. Biotechnological production of taxol and related taxoids: Current state and prospects. Anti-Cancer Agents in Medicinal Chemistry. 2009;**9**(1):109-121. DOI: 10.2174/187152009787047761

[65] Malik S, Cusidó RM, Mirjalili MH, Moyano E, Palazón J, Bonfill M. Production of the anticancer drug taxol in Taxus baccata suspension cultures: A review. Process Biochemistry. (Elsevier)

2011;**46**(1):23-34. DOI: 10.1016/j.procbio.2010.09.004

[66] Pan H et al. Repurposed antiviral drugs for COVID-19 – interim WHO SOLIDARITY trial results. medRxiv. 2020;**2**(1):5-10. DOI: 10.1101/2020.10.15.20209817

[67] Lem FF, Opook F, Lee DJH, Chee FT, Lawson FP, Chin SN. Molecular mechanism of action of repurposed drugs and traditional Chinese medicine used for the treatment of patients infected with COVID-19: A systematic scoping review. Frontiers in Pharmacology. 2021;**11**:2413. DOI: 10.3389/fphar.2020.585331

[68] WHO (World Health Organization). Anticipating Emerging Infectious Disease Epidemics. Geneva: WHO; 2015. Available from: https://apps.who.int/iris/bitstream/handle/10665/252646/WHO-OHE-PED-2016.2-eng.pdf

[69] WHO. WHO | What Is a Pandemic? Geneva: WHO; 2015. Available from: https:// www.who.int/csr/disease/swineflu/ frequently_asked_questions/pandemic/en/ [Accessed: December 30, 2018]

[70] Yu P, Hu B, Shi ZL, Cui J. Geographical structure of bat SARS-related coronaviruses. Infection, Genetics and Evolution. (Elsevier, B.V.) 2019;**69**:224-229. DOI: 10.1016/j.meegid.2019.02.001

[71] Delaune D et al. A novel SARS-CoV-2 related coronavirus in bats from Cambodia. Nature Communications. 2021;**12**(1):1-7. DOI: 10.1038/s41467-021-26809-4

[72] Li LL et al. A novel SARS-CoV-2 related coronavirus with complex recombination isolated from bats in Yunnan province, China. Emerging Microbes and Infections. 2021;**10**(1):1683-1690. DOI: 10.1080/22221751.2021.1964925/SUPPL_FILE/TEMI_A_1964925_SM3486.DOCX

[73] Zhou H et al. Identification of novel bat coronaviruses sheds light on the evolutionary origins of SARS-CoV-2 and related viruses CAS-TWAS Center of excellence for emerging infectious diseases (CEEID). bioRxiv. 2021;**2**(3):2021-2030 DOI: 10.1016/j.cell.2021.06.008

[74] Takashita E et al. Efficacy of antiviral agents against the SARS-CoV-2 omicron subvariant BA.2. New England Journal of Medicine. 2022;**386**(15):1475-1477. DOI: 10.1056/NEJMC2201933/SUPPL_FILE/NEJMC2201933_DISCLOSURES.PDF

[75] Pachetti M et al. Emerging SARS-CoV-2 mutation hot spots include a novel RNA-dependent-RNA polymerase variant. Journal of Translational Medicine. 2020;**18**(1):1-9. DOI: 10.1186/S12967-020-02344-6/FIGURES/4

[76] Zeng L, Li D, Tong W, Shi T, Ning B. Biochemical features and mutations of key proteins in SARS-CoV-2 and their impacts on RNA therapeutics. Biochemical Pharmacology. 2021;**189**:114424. DOI: 10.1016/J.BCP.2021.114424

[77] Cao Y et al. Omicron escapes the majority of existing SARS-CoV-2 neutralizing antibodies. Nature. 2021;**602**(7898):657-663. DOI: 10.1038/s41586-021-04385-3

[78] Tambunan USF, Fardiansyah Nasution MA, Alkaff AH. Introductory chapter: Application of peptides in biomedical sciences. In: Polypeptide - New

Insight into Drug Discovery and Development. London, UK: Intechopen; 2018. DOI: 10.5772/ INTECHOPEN.79297

[79] Wang C et al. A human monoclonal 1 antibody blocking SARS-CoV-2 infection. bioRxiv. 2020;**3**(1):22-32. DOI: 10.1101/2020.03.11.987958

[80] Shanmugaraj B, Siriwattananon K, Wangkanont K, Phoolcharoen W. Perspectives on monoclonal antibody therapy as potential therapeutic intervention for coronavirus disease-19 (COVID-19). Asian Pacific Journal of Allergy and Immunology. (NLM (Medline)) 2020;**38**(1):10-18. DOI: 10.12932/AP-200220-0773

[81] Fakih TM. ARTICLE HISTORY Dermaseptin-based antiviral peptides to prevent COVID-19 through In silico molecular docking studies against SARS-CoV-2 spike protein. Pharmaceutical Sciences and Research (PSR). 2020;**7**(4):65-70. Available from: http://www.rcsb.org/pdb

[82] Khaitov M et al. Silencing of SARS-CoV-2 with modified siRNA-peptide dendrimer formulation. Allergy. 2021;**00**:1-15. DOI: 10.1111/ALL.14850

[83] Åkerström S, Mirazimi A, Tan YJ. Inhibition of SARS-CoV replication cycle by small interference RNAs silencing specific SARS proteins, 7a/7b, 3a/3b and S. Antiviral Research. 2007;**73**(3):219-227. DOI: 10.1016/j.antiviral.2006.10.008

[84] Chowdhury UF, Sharif Shohan MU, Hoque KI, Beg MA, Sharif Siam MK, Moni MA. A computational approach to design potential siRNA molecules as a prospective tool for silencing nucleocapsid phosphoprotein and surface glycoprotein gene of SARS-CoV-2. Genomics. 2021;**113**(1):331-343. DOI: 10.1016/j.ygeno.2020.12.021

Section 2

Specific Cases Report

Chapter 2

Pluralism Medical Treatment, Prevention, and Control of COVID-19 Infection and Its Long-Sufferings among the Older Adults in the Northeast of Thailand from 2019 to 2022

Pissamai Homchampa, Khemika Napattaradechanon, Parichat Yatniyom, Thawalrat Ratanasiri, Piyaporn Sansila, Thanawan Sirisuk, Thawalwong Ratanasiri and Amornrat Ratanasiri

Abstract

COVID-19 in 2019 has brought both changes and challenges to the world. This global pandemic has an impact on people of all age levels, especially older adults. In Thailand, older persons are at high risk of COVID-19 infection. They are included in the so-called 608 groups. The objective of this review article was to synthesize and present medical pluralism, the development of drugs from herbs, and projects conducted to treat, prevent, and control the infection and long sufferings of COVID-19. The review covers 10 studies, three projects produced at Mahasarakham University, Chaiyaphum Rajabhat University, and Khon Kaen University that were reviewed, synthesized, and analyzed. The results of the synthesis indicate that modern and Thai traditional medicine can help reduce the severity of the infection and long sufferings of COVID-19. The medical pluralism between modern and Thai traditional medicine is needed to remedy COVID-19 cases among the older adults in the Northeast of Thailand.

Keywords: pluralism medical treatment, prevention and control, COVID-19 infection, long COVID-19 suffering, the Northeast of Thailand

1. Introduction

The global pandemic of COVID-19 has an impact on people of all age levels [1]. Similar to other countries, older adults are more likely to have a chronic illness [1].

Over the world reported that 66% of people aged 70 and over have at least one underlying condition that increased the risk of the severe impact of COVID-19 infection and its long sufferings [1].

The Ministry of Public Health (MOPH), the leader of the Department of Disease Control, nongovernmental organizations, and local organizations have an active role and follow the World Health Organization's (WHO's) eight pillars of COVID-19 response, which are a good guide for strengthening surveillance, case investigation, and the laboratory system, institutionalizing, the mechanism of coordination, and strengthening communication between stakeholders [1]. Medical pluralism (MP) is used for the treatment, prevention, and control of the COVID-19 pandemic in Thailand since 2019 [2–5].

The World Health Organization (WHO) acknowledges that Thailand shows significant progress on overall population health indicators, as seen in the relatively low COVID-19 cases number (less than one death per million population) and improving capacity for pandemic response [1]. WHO has recognized Thai Village Health Volunteers (VHVs) as "unsung heroes" who have made a great effort to fight COVID-19 [6]. The VHVs formulated "Socio-politics networks" or can be seen as a "Pluralistic network" based on a "collaborative system" between numerous agents/stakeholders in the community, including VHV groups, villagers, families/households level politicians' officials, and private sector actors [6, 7].

In the Northeast of Thailand, research and project produced by the staff of Mahasarakham University (MSU), Chaiyaphum Rajabhat University (CPRU), and Khon Kaen University (KKU) presented medical pluralism, development of herb medicine, health-seeking behaviors of older adults for treatment, prevention, and control of COVID-19 infection and its long sufferings [8–22].

This study aimed to synthesize knowledge about successful cases of pluralism medical treatment, prevention, and control of COVID-19 infection and its long sufferings among older adults.

2. Objective

The objective of this study was to synthesize knowledge about the successful pluralism of medical treatment, prevention, and control of COVID-19 infection and its long sufferings among the older population in the Northeast of Thailand from 2019 to 2022.

3. Methodologies

The study reviewed the results of the author's research and project in four steps as follows:

Step 1: Synthesize contents from the staff of Mahasarakham University (MSU), Chaiyaphum Rajabhat University (CPRU), and Khon Kaen University (KKU)'s research studies and projects from 1987 to 2022.

Step 2: Reported herbal medicine in pluralism medical treatment, prevention, and control of COVID-19 infection and its long COVID-19 sufferings.

Step 3: Reported cases of success in treatment, prevention, and control of COVID-19 infected.

Step 4: Summarized the organization chart related to the pluralism medical treatment in the Northeast of Thailand.

The research review was approved by the Ethics Committee for Human Research at Mahasarakham University (MSU), Chaiyaphum Rajabhat University (CPRU), and Khon Kaen University (KKU) (HE591125).

Most of the research studies were based on secondary data. Those who volunteered had signed the consent form.

4. Results

There are four steps to this research result as follows:

In step 1: We reviewed research results of pluralism medical treatment, prevention, and control of COVID-19 Infection and its long sufferings among the older adults. This study was analyzed and found that since 1987 the staff of Mahasarakham University (MSU), Chaiyaphum Rajabhat University (CPRU), and Khon Kaen University (KKU)'s research studies and projects about the elderly, promotion of herbal medicine gave knowledge of working with COVID-19 outbreaks since 2019 to health personnel by academic conference [8–22], as summarized in **Tables 1** and **2**.

For older adults, these three universities had worked with this problem to prepare health personnel to face aging as advancement in medical technology has resulted in the Thai population having a longer life expectancy, leading Thailand to the "Aging Society". Such changes affect the quality of life of the elderly and the working-age population who are direct caregivers. Ministry of Public Health prepares to step into a quality elderly society. The policy to promote the health of the elderly in the issue of "Long-term care for the elderly" to create understanding and ability to implement the policy appropriately.

The health promotion policy "Long-term care for the elderly" uses an analysis through cultural sensitivity aspects. The formulation process was divided into the five stages of policy formation, namely: (1) Policy Agenda Setting, (2) Policy Formulation, (3) Policy Implementation, (4) Evaluation Stage Policy, and (5) Policy Implementation.

The results of the analysis revealed that: (1) the policy arose from two major currents, namely the mainstream and the policy stream; (2) it was the government's policy with cultural sensitivity due to the policy transformation, taking into account the classification of the elderly into three groups (the home group, the social group, and the bed group). The policy implementation strategy is open to each sub-district to be able to develop an innovative long-term care system that takes into account the local context, community potential, and social costs [21]. Besides this, Chaiyaphum Rajabhat University (CPRU)'s staff has the arrangement of teaching nursing student's computer-assisted instruction (CAI).

The computer-assisted instruction (CAI) was selected for gerontological nursing lessons on Depression, Dementia, Parkinson's, and Geriatric assessment. Thirty third-year nursing students of the Faculty of Nursing at Chaiyaphum Rajabhat University were attending the gerontological nursing course. The lessons on Depression, Dementia, Parkinson, and Geriatric assessment were taught via Tutorial Instruction Pattern. The constructed CAI efficiency was 87/84 with an E.I. value of 0.7, higher than the

Study No.	Title	Ref.	Study design	Age group (Years old)	Sample size (sex) (Data from)	Findings	Year of pubn.
1. [N]	The causes of unpopularity of the traditional medicine	[8]	• Descriptive study • Document Analysis • In-depth-interview • Participant observation of traditional medicine treatment	Most of them were older adults	• 30 patients • 30 Thai Traditional Medicine Doctors • 4 Experts persons.	Five factors affecting unpopularity of the Traditional medicine are as follows: 1. Socio-economic status of TTMD 2. Poor curative efficiency 3. Teaching and education system of TTMD 4. Law of government health service system 5. New Technology of modern biomedicine	1987
2. [N]	The promotion of herbal planting for medical use and increasing household income to the villagers	[9]	• Action research study • Planting of 300 kg of Curcuma longa lion by 2 villagers and 4 households	Most of them were older populations	20 community leaders and health volunteers (VHVs) 20 Villagers 4 Households at Mooban Bausimma Tambon Non-udom Amphur Chumpae Khon Kaen province	• Coucuna Longa Linn planting in 4.96 square meters • Sell 633 kg to Phon Hospital • Villagers received 4431 Baths or 651 Baths/household/ 9 months • The villagers in Mooban Bausimma and others 5 nearby gain knowledge and experience of herbal planting for medical use	1992
3. [N]	The promotion of health care and health environment of target populations women, children, and aging people) at Mooban sum, Amphur Mahachanachai, Yasothorn	[10]	• Action Research by Using • Health Education • Health training • Health Check	• Woman • Children • Aging	• 51 Woman • 40 Children • 34 Aging • 40 Caregivers of the Children • 30 Caregivers of the older adults	After 1 month, 3 months, and 1-year follow-up found that the target populations, increase of 1. The effectiveness of self-care 2. Best experiences of caring for children and aging peoples 3. Better health status than before	1992

DOI: http://dx.doi.org/10.5772/intechopen.106339

Study No.	Title	Ref.	Study design	Age group (Years old)	Sample size (sex) (Data from)	Findings	Year of pubn.
						4. Need health team to evaluate sustainable development after 5 year	
4. [N]	The factors affecting an acceptance of herbal treatment	[11]	• Survey of knowledge, opinion, and experiment on 5 herbs in Thai Traditional Medicine (TTM) 1. Aloe 2. Snake plant 3. Candle bush 4. Curcuma longs Linn 5. Andrographis paniculate • Utilized TTM in Phon Hospital	18-85 years old mean age 51 74 Males 127 Females	OPD cases at Phon hospital 112 used modern Medicine and 89 cases used Thai Traditional Medicine (TTM)	77.1% present TTM equal to modern biomedicine 12.9% herbs better than modern biomedicine 76.6% herbs cheaper than modern drugs, factors affecting are as follows: 1. beliefs in herbal curative efficiency 2. receiving advice from the health personals 3. receiving advice from the relative's neighbor 4. receiving advice from mass media 5. physician-prescribed herbs for the patients	1995
5. [N]	The problems of seeking continuous medical care of patients with paralysis in Nonmuang Village, T. Sila, A. muang, Khon Kaen Province.	[12]	Descriptive study	All of them were older adults	11 cases living in Nonmuang village, Khon Kaen 5 Males 6 Females With hemiplegia caused by stroke, and had spinal cord disease	6 cases get better 2 cases stable 3 cases worsened • Three cases believe that they will remain stable • Four cases believe that they will get worse • One has no idea • Srinagarind Hospital and Nonmuang primary care unit has responsibility for continuous medical care	2005

Study No.	Title	Ref.	Study design	Age group (Years old)	Sample size (sex) (Data from)	Findings	Year of pubn.
6. [N]	Proportion of outpatient's perception in Srinagarind hospital about drugs after receiving from central dispensary	[13]	• Descriptive study • Using time allocation • Interviewed cases	18-84 years old median (45.6, IQR 18) 39.9% were educated as Bachelor's degree	143 cases at our outpatients at Srinagarind Hospital 44 Males 99 Females	• Half of them had the right drug perception • Factors that decreased drug perception were receiving new drugs and more amount of drugs	2016
7. [I]	Effect of institution-based management for elderly health promotion programs in Northeastern Thailand	[14]	• Interviewed • Clinical, diagnostic management • Examine IBM-EHP program	Older adults 60 years old and over	60 cases 55 controls	Cases demonstrated improvements in perceived self-efficacy, received social support, health promotion behavior, and HDL-C level ($p < 0.05$) than control	2016
8. [N]	Health promotion behaviors of elderly living in an urban community of Khon Kaen Province	[15]	Descriptive study	60-79 years old	545 older adults 218 Males 327 Females	Factors related to health promotion behaviors were as follows: 1. Caregiver at home 2. Home visit by a health care professional 3. Health promotion training 4. Health promotion education 5. Community broadcasting tower 6. Television and radio as $p < 0.05$	2018
9. [N]	Frailty and associated factors of elderly Buddhist monks in Chiang Mai Province, Thailand	[16]	• Cross-sectional descriptive study • Interviewed • Physical examination	Age 60 and over	135 older Buddhist monks	• 80.0% pre-frailty • 7.4% frailty Barthel ADL. Score 12 • 85.2% low grip strength • 17.8% Self-reported exhaustion • 17.0% Slow walking speed	2019

DOI: http://dx.doi.org/10.5772/intechopen.106339

Study No.	Title	Ref.	Study design	Age group (Years old)	Sample size (sex) (Data from)	Findings	Year of pubn.
						• 4.4% Low level of physical activity • 3.0% unintentional weight loss	
10. [I]	Health problems and health care outcomes of older patients admitted to intensive care units in the low and middle-income counties: A systematic and review meta-analysis	[17]	Systematic and review meta-analysis published from 2010 to 2019	• Older patients admitted to ICUs in the LMICS • Age 60 years old and over	10 out of 1486 observational studies from 4915 from 6 general and 13 specialty ICUs in the 7 LMICS	• Over one-fourth of older patients had severe conditions and loss of functional independence on ICU admission. • Infection-related problems were evidenced during ICU stays	2020

I: index journal; and N: non-index journal.

Table 1.
Summary of medical pluralism (MP) from MSU, CPRU, and KKU staffs' publications and presentations from 1987 to 2022.

Study No.	Title	Ref.	Study Design	Age group (years old)	Sample size (sex) (Data from)	Findings	Year of pubn.
1 [P]	Poster presentation: "Maelong volunteer for long-term care"	[18]	• Trained the health volunteers (VHVs) • Evaluated their knowledge, attitudes, and practices (KAP)	Most of them are adults and aging who work as VHVs at Maelong village	• 28 VHVs • 1 Male • 27 Females	• Increase awareness of long-term care • Gain more knowledge of caring for aging • Need repeat training every year	2018
2(AC)	The 1st Academic Conference "COVID-19 Situation Nursing Challenge", during 1-2 June 2021 at Faculty of Nursing, Chaiyaphum Rajabhat University, Chaiyaphum Province	[19]	Zoom Conference	Participants were 25 years old and over 60 years old	300 participants were Registered nurses who work in Thailand and abroad.	Most of them get more knowledge about the prevention and control of people and people infected with COVID-19 in terms of policy and practice	During 1-2 June 2021
3(AC)	The 2nd Academic Conference "COVID-19 Situation Leadership: Nursing Challenge", during 7-9 April 2022 at Faculty of Nursing, Chaiyaphum Rajabhat University, Chaiyaphum Province	[20]	Zoom Conference	Participants were 25 years old and over 60 years old	250 participants were Registered nurses who work in Thailand and abroad.	Most of them developed nursing leadership potential in the situation of COVID-19, covering services, administration, research, and nursing education.	During 7-9 April 2022

P: poster presentation; and AC: academic conference.

Table 2.
Summary of project related to the older populations and Medical Pluralism (MP) from MSU, CPRU, and KKU staffs' presentation during 2018-2022.

expected criteria. It was found that the mean score of the students' knowledge at post-test (x = 9.00) was higher than those at pre-test (x = 6.00), with a significant level of $p < 0.001$. Moreover, the score of satisfaction toward the CAI was high on every item. The computer-assisted instruction results in the student's acquiring knowledge on nursing care of gerontological nursing [22].

For giving knowledge of COVID-19 infected during the pandemic in 2019–2022, Chaiyaphum Rajabhat University (CPRU) had organized two academic conferences to educate professional nurses about the prevention and control of people and people infected with COVID-19 in terms of both policy and practice. Those professional nurses were provided with knowledge and understanding of situations and trends for the COVID-19 management. At the conference, the Director-General of the Department of Medical Sciences gave a talk on treating and caring for COVID-19 patients by medical professionals, effects and infection control in Asian countries including Japan and Indonesia, management for nurses in hospitals, roles of professional nurses in hospitals and communities, and application of nursing theories and processes. The conference was continually organized as the second meeting to develop nursing leadership potential in the situation of COVID-19. This second conference covered services, administration, research, and nursing education. The conference was paid an honor by the Dean of the Faculty of Nursing at UCLA and was attended by scholars from all the regions of Thailand and professional nurses who work in Thailand and abroad (**Table 2**).

In step 2: Reported herbal medicine in pluralism medical treatment, prevention, and control of COVID-19 infection and its long sufferings of Thai people in the Northeast of Thailand.

To promote herbal medicine, the staff of Khon Kaen University (KKU), Mahasarakham University (MSU), and Phon Hospital gave knowledge and practice to the villagers in Khon Kaen province. The results showed that the Community leaders, Health Volunteers (VHVs), and the villagers gain more knowledge and experience of herbal planting for medical use and increase household income (**Table 1**).

The medical practice guidelines, diagnosis, treatment, and prevention of infection in the hospital in case of Coronavirus infection in 2019 (COVID-19) from the Department of Thai Traditional and Alternative Medicine, Ministry of Public Health, the treatment of COVID-19 are as below:

Probable case person with test results positive for Rapid Antigen Test or Antigen Test Kit (ATK per SAR-CoV-2), and total confirmed cases, both those who have symptoms and asymptomatic person separate group according to the severity of the disease and risk factors can be in four cases as follows:

1. Asymptomatic COVID-19

    - Out-patients with self-isolation, home isolation, or state locations are provided as appropriate
    - Provide symptomatic care
    - Do not give antiviral drugs such as Favipiravir due to most of the patients' s symptoms decreasing on their own.
    - Consider giving Andrographis paniculate for treatment
    - Do not give Andrographis paniculate with an antiviral drug, because there may be side effects from the medicine.

2. Symptomatic COVID-19 without pneumonia, and no risk factors for severe disease.

    - May consider giving Favipiravir by starting the drug as soon as possible.

- If the infection is detected when the patient has symptoms for more than 5 days and the patient is asymptomatic, or the patient had few symptoms, may not need to give the antiviral drug, because the patient may heal by themselves without the complications.

3. COVID-19 with mild symptoms, but has risk factors for severe disease or having comorbidity or mild pneumonia, any of the risk factors are as follows:

    - Older than 60 years
    - Chronic Obstructive Pulmonary Disease (COPD), includes another Chronic Lung Disease
    - Chronic Kidney Disease (CKD)
    - Cardiovascular disease, including congenital heart disease
    - Cerebrovascular disease
    - Uncontrollable Diabetes
    - Obesity (weight more than 90 Kg, or BMI > 30 Kg/Square meter)
    - Liver Cirrhosis
    - Low immunity, and lymphocytes less than 1000 cells/cubic millimeter, or
    - Patients without risk factors, but tends to the severity of the disease increased

It is recommended to use only one antiviral drug as below, considering congenital disease; contraindications to the drug against each other of antivirus drug, and original medicine (drug-drug interaction), bed management, ease of drug administration, and reserve dose of drugs.

1. Nirmatrelvir/ritonavir for 5 days (Medication is not recommended, if systems last more than 5 days), or.
2. Molnupiravir for 5 days (This medication is not recommended for use if symptoms persist for more than 7 days).
3. Remdesivir for 3 days (This medication is not recommended for use if symptoms persist for more than 7 days).
4. Favipiravir for 5–10 days (This medication is not recommended for use if symptoms persist for more than 4 days).

4. Confirmed patients with pneumonia, who have hypoxia (resting oxygen saturation <94%), or have hypoxia (SPO2 > 3%) of measured value while

exercising (exercise-induced hypoxemia) or chest radiograph has the progression of pulmonary infiltrates.

- Recommend Remdesivir for 5–10 days, in the patients who require oxygen, depending on the clinical symptom, the patients should closely follow-up for the symptoms.

- First choice, in the case of mild pneumonia at SpO2 during 94-96%, or no oxygen receives, may consider giving Molnupiravir for 5 days, which should start using the drug within 5 days, after symptoms or Remdesivir, which gives within 7 days after symptoms.

- Consider giving Remdesivir for 5–10 days as follows:

    - Patients with mild symptoms but their risk factors for the severe disease, or have major comorbidities or patients with pneumonia, also do not need oxygen.

    - Patients with severe pneumonia no later than 10 days after symptoms, and receive cannula >1 liter/min, and level of SpO2 < 95%, or receive HFNC/NIVHFNC or use a ventilator (if wear a breathing apparatus may benefit from this drug is not fully).

    - Pregnant woman with pneumonia (has more details on the topic of treatment COVID-19 in pregnant women).

    - There are contraindications to the administration of the drug by mouth or absorption problems.

- Choose to use antiviral drugs, kind to eat or Remdesivir, either not shared due to medicine active in the same position when giving Remdesivir until the recommended date.

- No recommend Corticosteroid in case of mild symptoms (No additional oxygen is required), or asymptomatic pneumonia.

The Department of Thai Traditional and Alternative Medicine presented the restored health after COVID-19 infection with herbal medicine as shown in **Table 3**.

In step 3: We reported case success in treatment prevention and control of COVID-19 infected.

Since 2019, the elderly who get COVID-19 received treatment in the hospital and home isolation. The older adults who used medical pluralism (MP) during treatment were our case studies.

We followed the treatment of Coronavirus with the phone who was admitted to the University Hospital of KKU and MSU. Those cases who did not use MP and died from their complication did not report in this study.

We could only review report the number of cases with COVID-19 on May 31, 2022 at the Area Health District, which includes seven provinces in the Northeast of

Herbal medicine name	Properties
Andrographis panicolata	Reduce fever, anti-inflammatory
Benjalokwichian Medicine	Cure a fever, make poison out of the body
Prasacanthr Daeng Medicine (Dracaena loureiroi Gagnep)	Reduce fever, hot fix, cure thirst
Reduce Fever Medicine namely Junleera	Relieve symptoms of fever, seasonal Fever
Aromatic Medicine namely Na Wa Kot	Cure wind dizziness, Squeamish, vomit, fix the wind, late fever
Triphala	Cough relief, expectorant, Elemental balance
Cough Medicine namely Makhampom	Expectorant, cough relief
Ginger pill	Relieve flatulence, and indigestion, expel cure heartburn
Cannabidial (CBD oil)	Cure insomnia, headache, and appetizing
Muscle Relaxants	Joint pain relief, muscle pain chest pain, stomach ache
Ya SUK SAI YAI	Cure insomnia, for mode changes, alleviate exhaustion

Source: Department of Thai Traditional and Alternative Medicine, 2022.

Table 3.
Restore health after COVID-19 Infection with herbal medicine (Available from: https://web.facebook.com/informationcovid19/posts/498540561764273?_rdc=1&_rdr).

Thailand such as Udon Thani, Sakon Nakhon, Nakhon Phanom. Loei, Nong Khai, Nong Bua Lamphu, and Bueng Kan reported cases of COVID-19 as +264 new cases; 123,760 cumulative patients, 21,956 hospitalized, and 120,195 healed [23].

Our cases reported from 2019 to 2022 are divided into four groups as follows:

1. Case of unable to COVID vaccination

2. Case of COVID-19 infected

3. Case of COVID-19 infection and its long-sufferings

4. Case of the older adults' health-seeking behavior in the Northeast of Thailand during COVID-19 Outbreaks

4.1 Case of unable to COVID vaccination

One Thai male, age 64 years old who cannot vaccinate COVID vaccine since 2019, because he has health problems of chronic illness and heart diseases. He needs to insert three catheters entering the heart and used much medicine to protect against embolism. His life is very difficult during the COVID-19 pandemic in Thailand.

He changes his lifestyle by quitting smoking, taking medicine and food as prescribed by the doctor, taking some supplements and herbs, exercising according to the doctor's orders, living in a well-ventilated environment, getting enough rest, and following Thai policies to prevent COVID-19 infection. He insisted that pluralism of medical treatment prevention and control of COVID-19 infection was very good for him.

4.2 Case of COVID-19 infected

One Thai female, age 70 years old who had controllable diabetes mellitus, got COVID-19 infected with test results positive for Rapid Antigen Test. She was asymptomatic COVID-19 and received Andrographis Paniculate for treatment and home isolation. She takes this medicine and food as prescribed by the doctor, exercises according to the doctor's order, lives in a well-ventilated environment, and gets enough rest.

Nowadays, she takes some supplements and herbs, also has health practices as above, and follows Thai policies to prevent long Covid-19 suffering.

4.3 Case of COVID-19 infection and its long sufferings

One Thai female, age 59 years old, got COVID-19 infected in 2021 with symptomatic COVID-19 without pneumonia and no risk factors for severe disease. Her doctor gave Favipiravir by starting the drug as soon as possible. But she needs to work hard and not get enough rest.

At present, she still has a persistent cough. She uses cough medicine, namely Makhampom for cough relief, takes some supplement and herbs, and follows Thai policies to prevent COVID-19 infected to other people nearby.

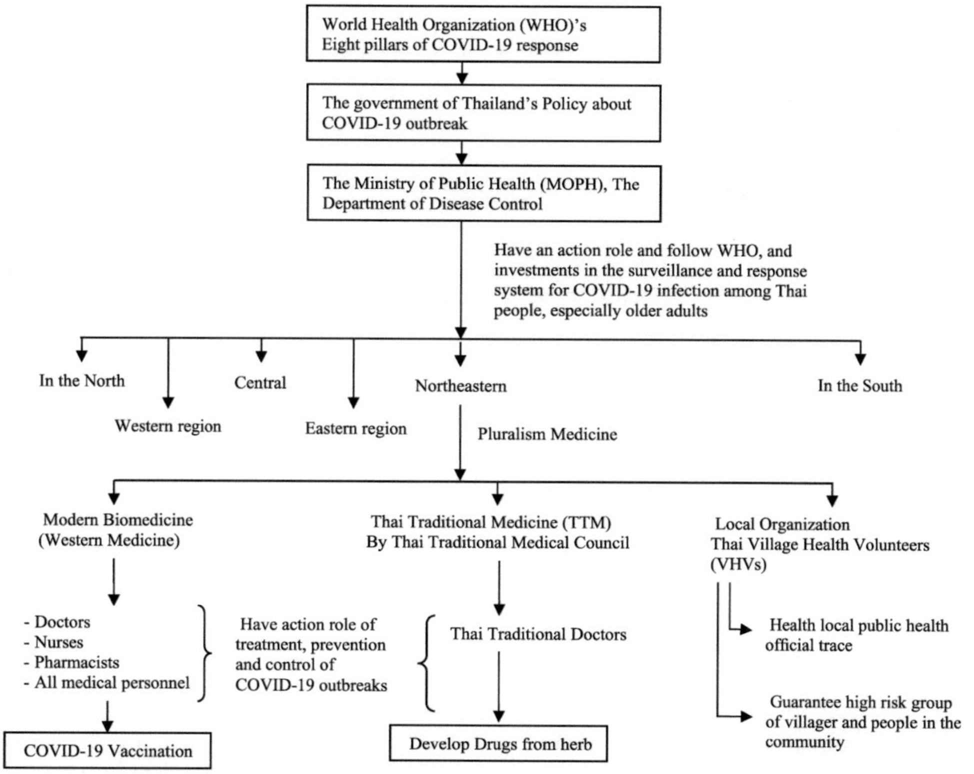

Figure 1.
Summarized the organization chart related to pluralism medical treatment in Northeastern, Thailand, since 2019.

4.4 Case of the older adults' health-seeking behavior in the Northeast of Thailand during COVID-19 Outbreaks

One Thai female, age 60 years old, she fell in the bathroom and ruptured blood vessels in the brain that paralyzed her. Her husband is famous for Thai traditional treatment, but her daughter believes in treatment with modern medicine because she works in one private hospital in Khon Kaen province. During the COVID-19 outbreak in Thailand, patients have difficulty going to the hospital.

Her family members always quarreled about treatment. One female health volunteer in this village recommended her family and other patients to the treatment of Thai traditional medicine and modern medicine. After that, this older adult with hemiplegia gradually got better, and her family is happy.

In step 4: We summarized the organization chart related to pluralism medical treatment in Northeastern, Thailand, since 2019.

Medical pluralism (MP) plays a role in many people's lives over the world. Older people in the Northeast of Thailand are familiar with the herb, Thai government policies have implemented pluralism medicine for treatment, prevention, and control of COVID-19 infected Thai people as summarized by the organization as present in **Figure 1**.

5. Discussions

Medical pluralism (MP) is used in many countries over the world during the COVID-19 outbreak. Our review articles found that pluralism in medical treatment, prevention, and control of COVID-19 infection and its long sufferings was found in most older adults worldwide, it presented that most countries have medical pluralism (MP) for care sickness of the populations [24].

The government of Thailand focuses on the older adults and classified them as a risk group, by giving it the name 608 groups (groups of people who need to get vaccinated with the most COVID are older people aged 60 years and over and those with underlying disease, including chronic respiratory disease, cardiovascular disease, chronic renal disease, cerebrovascular disease, obesity, cancer, and diabetes) that will be vaccinated in the first priority group. Similar to other countries, which are the aging society, they also focus on the older populations, they arranged at least three vaccinations of COVID-19 vaccine for those older adults [25].

Most Thai older adults are familiar with herbs because it's grown for food and medicine [9, 11]. During the COVID-19 outbreak in 2019, Thai older people in rural communities used herbs, such as Andrographis paniculate to build immunity for preventing COVID-19 infection [26]. Similar to other studies presented, herbal medicine is a class of natural substances and is also used as adjuvant therapy for COVID-19. These herbal medicines are psoralidine, silverstrol, quwrrectin, myricellin, flavonoids, and polyphenols [27–29].

Health interventions have been implemented, reducing the rate of the COVID-19 infection, including a face mask, hand hygiene, COVID vaccination, home isolation, and social distancing, similar to the prior studies [30, 31].

Our review of research, and projects produced at Mahasarakham University (MSU), Chaiyaphum Rajabhat University (CPRU), and Khon Kaen University (KKU) presented that Modern Biomedicine and Thai Traditional Medicine can help reduce the severity of the infection and long sufferings of the COVID-19 during 2019–2022, among the older adults in the Northeast of Thailand.

6. Conclusion

The medical pluralism (MP) between modern biomedicine and Thai traditional medicine is needed to remedy COVID-19 cases among the older adults because most of them are familiar with herbs used in their household for food and medicine.

The promotion of herbal planting for medical use, which is increasing household income for the villagers in the Northeast of Thailand, should be widely developed and safe for all people in Thailand.

Acknowledgements

The authors thank (a) all the respondents for their valuable contribution to this study, (b) The Faculty of Medicine of Mahasarakham University and Khon Kaen University for data and financial support, (c) The Faculty of Nursing of Chaiyaphum Rajabhat University for data and financial support, and (d) Dr. Thawalsak Ratanasiri, Dr. Bangonsri Jindawong, Dr. Chanchanok Aramrat, and Mrs. Sompong Chantakram for help search.

Conflict of interest

All authors declare that they have no conflicts of interest.

Author details

Pissamai Homchampa[1], Khemika Napattaradechanon[2], Parichat Yatniyom[2], Thawalrat Ratanasiri[3], Piyaporn Sansila[1], Thanawan Sirisuk[4], Thawalwong Ratanasiri[3] and Amornrat Ratanasiri[5]*

1 Faculty of Medicine, Mahasarakham University, Mahasarakham, Thailand

2 Faculty of Nursing, Chaiyaphum Rajabhat University, Chaiyaphum, Thailand

3 Faculty of Medicine, Khon Kaen University, Khon Kaen, Thailand

4 Private Clinic in Bangkok, Bangkok, Thailand

5 Faculty of Medicine, Department of Community Medicine, Khon Kaen University, Khon Kaen, Thailand

*Address all correspondence to: amorat@kku.ac.th

References

[1] Agartan TI, Cook S, Lin V. Introduction: COVID-19 and WHO: Global institutions in the context of shifting multilateral and regional dynamics. Global Social Policy. 2020; **20**(3):367-373

[2] Muangsakul W, Srisuantang S, Sajjasophon R. Medical pluralism for community health in Thammasen sub-district, Photharam District, Ratchaburi province, Thailand. Journal of Health Research. 2018;**32**(4):313-321

[3] Cant S. Medical pluralism, mainstream marginality or subaltern therapeutics? Globalization and the integration of 'Asian' medicines and biomedicine in the UK. Society and Culture in South Asia. 2020;**6**(1): 31-51

[4] Leslie C. Medical pluralism in world perspective. Social Science & Medicine. Part B. Medical Anthropology. 1980; **14**(4):191-195

[5] Foran BJ. Medical Pluralism and Global Health Policy: The Integration of Traditional Medicine in Health Care Systems. University of Western Sydney (Australia); 2007. pp. 1-378. Available from: https://researchdirect.westernsydney.edu.au.islandora/object/yws.3623. (Accessed: May 10, 2022)

[6] Jiaviriyaboonya P. Anthropological study of village health volunteers' (VHVs') socio-political network in minimizing risk and managing the crisis during COVID-19. Heliyon. 2022;**8**(1): e08654

[7] United Nations Thailand. Social Impact Assessment of COVID-19 in Thailand. Oxford Policy Management Limited; 2020. pp. 1-176. Available from: www.opml.co.uk [Accessed: June 9, 2022]

[8] Supasilapa S, Sinsuphan N, Ratanasiri A. The causes of unpopularity of the traditional medicine. Srinagarind Hospital Medical Journal. 1987;**2**(3): 182-190

[9] NaNakorn S, Iamwiriyawat S, Ratanasiri A, Doiwnsodsai P, Kessomboon P, Sansila P, et al. The promotion of herbal planting for medical use and increasing household income to the villagers. Khon Kaen Agriculture Journal. 1992;**20**(3):153-161

[10] Ratanasiri A, Sri-akjunt N, Homchampa P, NaNakorn S, Kesomboon P, Ditstapornncharoen W, et al. The promotion of health care and health environment of target populations (women, children and aging person) at Mooban Sum, Amphur Mahachanachai, Yasothorn Province. Khon Kaen Agriculture Journal. 1992;**20**(4):213-221

[11] NaNakorn S, Ratanasiri A, Sansila P, Kumsuk K. The factors affecting an acceptance of herbal treatment. Srinagarind Hospital Medical Journal. 1995;**10**(4):151-161

[12] Delake T, Patanawong P, Puttimatee N, Pudtanaratanamoree R, Sinsupan N, Ratanasiri A, et al. The problems of seeking continuous medical care of patients with paralysis in nonmuang village T.sila A.muang Khon Kaen Province. Srinagarind Medical Journal. 2005;**20**(4):202-207

[13] Kongtong T, Saengmongkonpipat P, Jeerasuwannakul W, Suwanchai K, Kuhirunyaratn P, Ratanasiri A, et al. Proportion of outpatient's perception in Srinagarind hospital about drugs after receiving from central dispensary. Srinagarind Medical Journal. 2016;**31**(5): 82-85

[14] Sombateyotha K, Pichainarong N, Schelp FP, Homchampa P. Effect of institution-based management for elderly health promotion program in Northeastern Thailand. The Southeast Asian Journal of Tropical Medicine and Public Health. 2016;**47**(5): 1062-1088

[15] Kuhirunyarath P, Ratanasiri A, Jindawong B, Natiboot P, Watchanapan L, Junthakhun C, et al. Health promotion behaviors of elderly living in an urban community of Khon Kaen Province. Srinagarind Medical Journal. 2018;**33**(2):153-160

[16] Ratanasiri T, Lerttrakarnnon P. Frailty and associated factors of elderly Buddhist monks in Chiang Mai Province, Thailand. Chiang Mai Medical Journal. 2019;**58**(4):211-221

[17] Le Lam TD, Homchampa P. Health problems and health care outcomes of older patients admitted to intensive care units in the low- and middle-income countries: A systematic and review meta-analysis. BJM. 2020;7(2):39-64

[18] Ratanasiri T. Poster Presentation of the Community Project title "Maelong Voleenteer Health Services are Fascinatingly and Dependable Project" under the supervision of Assoc. Prof. Dr. Peerasak Lerttrakarnnon, and Dr.Krid Thongbunjob for Family Medicine Study. Chiang Mai University, Chiang Mai, Thailand. 2018

[19] Napattaradechanon K, Yatniyom P. The 1st Academic Conference "COVID-19 Situation Nursing Challenge", during 1-2 June 2021 at Faculty of Nursing, Chaiyaphum Rajabhat University, Chaiyaphum Province

[20] Napattaradechanon K, Yatniyom P. The 2nd Academic Conference "COVID-19 Situation Leadership: Nursing Challenge", during 7-9 April 2022 at Faculty of Nursing, Chaiyaphum Rajabhat University, Chaiyaphum Province

[21] Yatniyom P, Loskultong P. An analysis of public policy on cultural sensitivity and health promotion for the elderly. Yuparat Jay. 2014;**4**(1):68-79

[22] Yatniyom P, Lalun A, Plairahan S, Mungkamanee S. Effects of Computer-assisted Instruction on Gerontological Nursing of Nursing students. Faculty of Nursing, Chaiyaphum Rajabhat University. Journal of the Royal Thai Army Nurses. 2020;**20**(3):411-421

[23] Area Health District 8 Situation report of COVID-19 in 2022. Available from: https://r8way.moph.go.th/r8way/covid-19 [Accessed: May 31, 2022]

[24] Tilburt JC, Miller FG. Responding to medical pluralism in practice: A principle ethical approach. Journal of American Board of Family Medicine. 2007;**20**(5): 489-494

[25] Yi M, Marathe A. Fairness versus efficiency of vaccine allocation strategies. Value in Health. 2015;**18**(2): 278-283

[26] Director General of the Department of Thai Traditional and Alternative Medicine. Division of Complementary and Alternative Medicine. Health Care Guidelines of Thai Traditional Medicine for COVID-19 patients. 1st edition. Bangkok: NSS Creation Limited; 2022. Available from: https://www.dtam.moph.go.th/index.php/en/department/psdg/42-download/8630-dl0130.html (Accessed: May 18, 2022)

[27] Artia YA, Alagawany MH, Farag MR, Alkhath FM, Khafaga AF, Abdel-Moneim AM, et al. Phytogenic products and phytochemicals a candidate strategy

to improve tolerance to coronavirus. Frontiers in Veterinary Science. 2020;**7**: 573159

[28] Guler HI, Talar G, Yildiz O, Belduz AO, Kolayil S. Investigation of potential inhibitors properties of ethanolic propolis extracts against ACE II receptors for COVID-19 treatment by molecular docking study. Archives of Microbiology. 2021;**203**(6):3557-3564

[29] Khayrani AC, Irdiani R, Aditama R, Pratami DK, Lischer K, Ansari MJ, et al. Evaluating the potency of Sulawesi propolis compounds as ACE-2 inhibitors through molecular docking for COVID-19 drug discovery preliminary study. Journal of King Saud University - Science. 2021;**33**(2):101297

[30] Department of Thai Traditional and Alternative Medicine. Division of Complementary and Alternative Medicine, Ministry of Public Health. Medical Practice guidelines, diagnosis, treatment, prevention and control of coronavirus infected in 2019. Available from: https://thaicam.go.th/ [Accessed October 26, 2021]

[31] Saghir SAM, Algabri NA, Alagawany MM, Artia YA, Alyleih SR, Ernest SS, et al. Chloroquine and hydroxychloroquine for the prevention and treatment of COVID-19: A fiction, hope or hype? An updated review. Therapeutics and Clinical Risk Management. 2021;**17**:371-387

Chapter 3

Baricitinib in the Treatment of COVID-19

Shubham Atal, Ananyan Sampath, Aditya Banerjee and Ratinder Jhaj

Abstract

Baricitinib is a novel Janus kinase (JAK) inhibitor which has recently been included in recommendations for treatment of COVID-19. This chapter is focused on discussing the evidence available regarding the safety and efficacy of use of baricitinib alone or in combination with other therapies for treatment of patients with COVID-19. A systematic literature search was conducted for this purpose to find all clinical studies on baricitinib in treatment of COVID-19. A total of 30 studies, including both clinical trials and observational studies were identified, and they have been described briefly. Collation of the results from these observational and interventional studies shows that baricitinib either alone or in combination with other drugs, when used as an add-on to standard therapy, was found to have favorable outcomes in hospitalized patients with moderate to severe COVID-19. Furthermore, ongoing clinical trials indicate that the drug is still under evaluation across the world for its safety and efficacy in COVID-19. The recent approval of baricitinib by the US FDA for treatment of hospitalized adults with COVID-19 accurately reflects the role of the drug in COVID-19. Baricitinib improves clinical outcomes in hospitalized COVID-19 patients, and additional evidence may establish the drug as a standard treatment in such patients.

Keywords: JAK kinase inhibitor, baricitinib, COVID-19, SARS-Cov-2, clinical outcomes, mortality

1. Introduction

Since causing an outbreak of a cluster of cases of pneumonia in Wuhan, China, the novel corona virus, named Severe Acute Respiratory Syndrome Coronavirus-2 (SARS-CoV-2), has spread globally to become one of the worst pandemics ever seen by humankind [1, 2]. With multiple 'waves' of the Corona Virus Disease known as COVID-2019 engulfing the world, the medical and scientific communities have focused their efforts on developing effective management strategies especially for hospitalized patients. These efforts have mostly been concentrated on evaluating the antiviral and anti-inflammatory properties of novel or repurposed medications. COVID-19 treatment guidelines from the World health Organization (WHO), the National Institutes of Health (NIH), U.S., the National Institute for Health and Care

Excellence (NICE), UK, and regional healthcare authorities such as Indian Council of Medical Research (ICMR) focus on the management of complications, the prevention of progression, and the provision of supportive care with symptomatic treatment based on evidence-based recommendations. A wide variety of clinical trials and observational studies have been conducted worldwide to evaluate treatment effects on survival rates in various severities of COVID-19 patients, as well as to reduction in morbidity in terms of hospitalization, time to recovery, and symptomatic or virological response in patients with less severe illness. COVID-19 treatments still remain limited; include antiviral therapies such as remdesivir, nirmatrelvir-ritonavir, molupiravir, immunomodulators such as corticosteroids, IL-6 inhibitors, and, more recently, specific monoclonal antibodies such as REGN-COV2 (casirivimab and imdevimab combination), regdanvimab, and sotrovimab among others [3–5].

The FDA granted emergency use authorization (EUA) to baricitinib, a novel Janus kinase (JAK) inhibitor, to be used in combination with remdesivir in November 2020 [6], which was later revised to a standalone therapy in adults and children above 2 years of age hospitalized for COVID-19 [7]. Finally, in May 2022, baricitinib has received approval from the FDA for the treatment of COVID-19 in hospitalized adults requiring supplemental oxygen, non-invasive or invasive mechanical ventilation, or extracorporeal membrane oxygenation (ECMO) [8]. At present, European Medicines Agency (EMA) is evaluating the marketing authorization application for baricitinib to be used in COVID-19 treatment protocol for patients above the age of 10 years of age who require supplemental oxygen therapy [9]. In May 2021, the Central Drugs Standard Control Organization (CDSCO), drug regulatory authority of India also granted emergency use approval to baricitinib for the treatment of confirmed COVID-19 hospitalized adults requiring supplemental oxygen in combination with remdesivir [10]. Baricitinib is an oral JAK 1 and 2 inhibitor that was approved for rheumatoid arthritis in the United States and Japan in 2017 [11]. JAKs are a family of enzyme involved in the inflammatory pathway that helps regulate the signaling cascade, activating signal transducers and activators of transcription (STATs) for cytokines such as IL-2, 6, 10, 12, IFN- etc. JAK inhibitors (JAK i's) have been shown to be clinically useful in immune, inflammatory, and hematopoietic diseases by preventing the dysregulated production of proinflammatory cytokines involved in cellular survival, proliferation, differentiation, and immigration [12, 13]. As a result, baricitinib has been studied in the treatment of COVID-19 with the goal of suppressing the hyperinflammatory state of cytokine release syndrome (CRS) or hypercytokinemia (cytokine storm) associated with COVID-19 [14].

Systematic/living reviews of COVID-19 therapies [15, 16] and JAK inhibitors [17, 18] are available. This chapter solely focuses on a comprehensive synthesis of the evidence available regarding use of baricitinib in treatment of COVID-19. For this purpose, we have used a systematic search strategy as recommended per the Cochrane methodology.

Figure 1 provides a schematic representation of the mechanism of action of Baricitinib, mainly on three different aspects of Corona Virus Disease, inhibits viral entry, inhibits Inflammation by blocking JAK–STAT signal transduction pathways and alters the immune status via JAK–STAT inhibition.

1.1 Search methodology

Literature search was conducted to identify studies which assess the efficacy and safety of baricitinib therapy in COVID-19, either alone or in combination with other therapies. This included interventional studies (Randomized Controlled Trials i.e.,

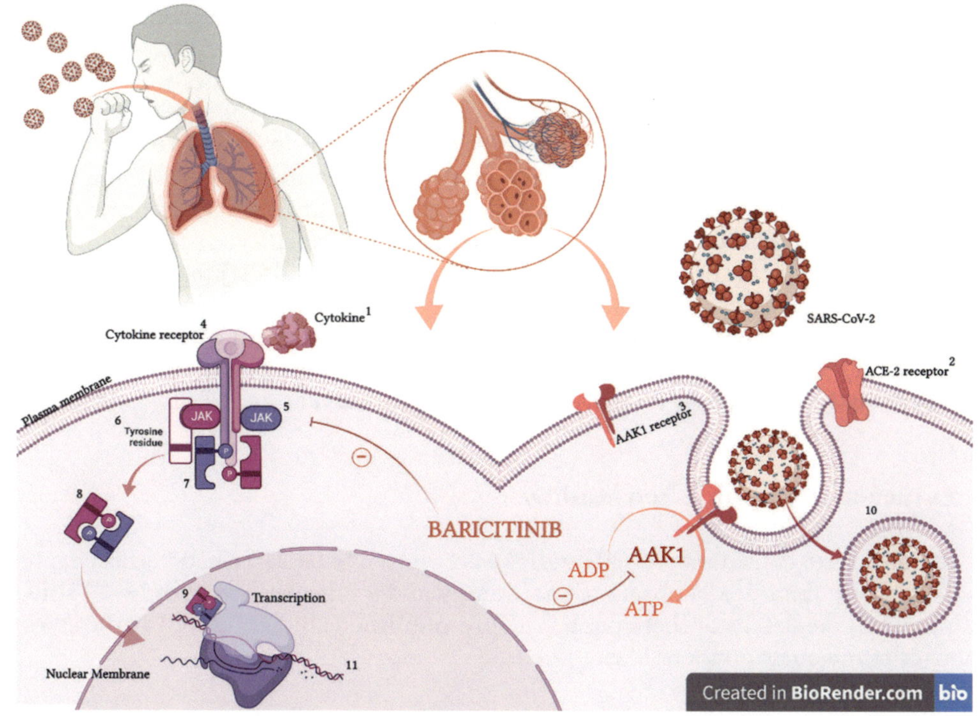

Figure 1.
Schematic representation of the mechanism of action of Baricitinib. [1] Interleukins (IL-2, IL-4, IL-7, IL-g, IL-15, IL-21, IL-6) are the most common. Baricitinib inhibits IL-2, IL-4, IL-7, IL-15, IL-21 via JAK1/3 STAT1/3/5 to regulate hemostasis and lymphocyte I proliferation, whereas IL6 acts via tyrosine kinase JAKl/2 STAT3 to regulate T cell differentiation and inflammation. [2] Angiotensin-ACE-2 receptor converting enzyme-2 functions as a docking receptor for SARS CoV-2 attachment. [3] AAKl-adaptor-associated protein I (AAKl-API). [4] Kinase I (AP2-associated protein kinase 1) is a transmembrane enzyme that participates in clathrin-mediated endocytosis. Baricitinib inhibits enzyme activation and thus prevents SARS-CoV 2 endocytosis. [4] Cytokine, type I and type II receptors. [5] Janus activated kinases are intracellular non-receptor tyrosine kinases that regulate cytokine signaling via the JAK–STAT pathway. Baricitinib is a JAK inhibitor that is not selective. [6] Tyrosine residues that aid in the binding of SH2 domain proteins like STAT. [7] Signal transduction activated transcription (STAT) is a downstream transducer of the JAK enzyme that exists intracellularly in an inactivated hypophosporylated state in association with JAK. [8] STAT phosphorylated active form. [9] Specific gene transcription activation. [10] Transcription is followed by protein translation, which results in the regulated effects.

RCTs and non RCTs) as well as observational studies assessing the efficacy and/or safety of baricitinib in COVID-19, published or pre-published (in English language) after December 2019. Case reports, review articles, conference proceedings, editorial/comments, author response or book chapter were not included.

The WHO COVID-19 Database (WHO COVID-19 Global literature on Coronavirus Disease) was used which is a comprehensive database of COVID-19 research articles [19] containing global literature from all major standard electronic databases of published, pre-published and gray literature sources such as MEDLINE, Scopus, ProQuest Central, ELSEVIER, Web of Science, EMBASE, ScienceDirect, CINAHL, CAB Abstracts, APA PsycInfo, ChemRxiv, BioMed Central, Oxford Academic, medRxiv, BMC, bioRxiv, etc. Furthermore, a manual search was performed using the bibliography of selected articles, and any studies that satisfied eligibility criteria were added. We searched all information sources up to May 31, 2022.

The list of keywords searched in the Titles, Abstracts and Authors, using Boolean operators consisted of *Baricitinib, Janus Kinase, JAK–STAT, Therapy, Treatment*,

2019 novel Coronavirus disease, COVID-19, SARS-CoV-2, novel Coronavirus infection, 2019-ncov infection, Coronavirus disease 2019, Coronavirus disease-19, 2019-ncov disease, COV, Coronavirus. After removing the duplicate results, the titles and abstracts were independently screened by two sets of reviewers based on the eligibility criteria and then assessed for availability of full texts. Data was then extracted from eligible studies related to pre-decided data items—study characteristics, patient characteristics, interventions studied, and outcomes reported. Standard definitions were used for the severity of disease and various outcome parameters [20].

We used the Cochrane tool for randomized trials (RoB 2.0) [21] to categorize the published RCTs as either low risk of bias, some concerns—probably low risk of bias, more concerns—probably high risk of bias, or high risk of bias. The "Study Quality Assessment tool" [22] was used for critical appraisal of internal validity and bias in observational studies (Non-Randomized Studies of Intervention, NRSIs).

2. Evidence from published studies

After careful consideration, 30 studies were chosen to be described in this chapter. Among these, there are 24 observational studies and 6 interventional studies. **Table 1** summarizes the details of these published/pre-published studies, as well as the assessment of study quality/risk of bias.

2.1 Observational studies

In a prospective cohort study conducted in Bangladesh, Hasan et al. [23] included 238 patients with severe COVID-19 pneumonia, 122 of whom received baricitinib 8 mg (high dose) and 116 patients received 4 mg (usual dose) orally for 14 days, along with dexamethasone, remdesivir, and enoxaparin/dalteparin. The time to achieve ≥94% oxygen saturation (5 vs 8 days; IQR: 4–5 and 6–9 days respectively, $P < 0.05$) and the need for supplemental oxygen were significantly shorter in the high dose group. Similarly, the need for intensive care unit (ICU) and intubation support was significantly lower in patients receiving the high dose of baricitinib compared to those receiving the usual dose (9 vs 17.2%, $P = 0.02$; 4.1 vs 9%, $P = 0.001$, respectively), as was the 30-day all-cause mortality (3.3 vs 6%, $P = 0.001$). The median duration of hospitalization in the high dose group was also shorter (11 vs 13 days; IQR: 9.5–14 and 10–17.5 days, respectively, $P = 0.072$). Thrombocytopenia and mouth sores were also significantly higher in the high dose group (9.8 vs 2.6% and 2.4 vs 0.8%, respectively). High-dose baricitinib treatment provided significant benefits in terms of survival and other clinical outcomes among patients with severe COVID-19, albeit at a higher risk of thrombocytopenia and mouth sores. The study participants, however, differed in clinical and biochemical parameters at baseline.

The same investigators conducted another prospective study involving 37 adult patients; 17 were assigned to the 'control' (No Loading Dose, NLD) group, while 20 were assigned to the 'case' (Loading Dose, LD) group, where they received an additional 8 mg loading dose of baricitinib orally before receiving 4 mg daily oral baricitinib for 14 days. Tolerability was good in both groups and there were no significant differences in mortality. However, the median time (in days) to reach $SpO_2 > 95\%$ was relatively shorter in the LD group as compared to NLD [3 (IQR:2–8) vs 4 (IQR:4–5) respectively, $P = 0.180$]. A similar trend was observed for the median time to return to normal breathing [(LD 5(4–5) vs NLD 8 (7–10) days] and the median time spent in the hospital (LD 12 vs NLD

S. N.	Title of study	Authors	Study location	Study design	Bias assessment
Observational studies					
1	Impact of high dose of baricitinib in severe COVID-19 pneumonia: a prospective cohort study in Bangladesh.	Hasan MJ, Rabbani R, Anam AM, Huq SM, Polish MM, Nessa SS, et al.	Bangladesh	Prospective Cohort	*Good*
2	Additional baricitinib loading dose improves clinical outcome in COVID-19	Hasan MJ, Rabbani R, Anam AM, Huq SM, Polash MM, Nessa SS, et al.	Bangladesh	Case Control	*Good*
3	Use of baricitinib in patients with moderate to severe Coronavirus Disease 2019	Titanji BK, Farley MM, Mehta A, Connor-Schuler R, Moanna A Cribbs SK, et al.	United States	Retrospective Cohort	*Fair*
4	Baricitinib restrains the immune dysregulation in patients with severe COVID-19.	Bronte V, Ugel S, Tinazzi E, Vella A, Sanctis FD, Canè S, et al.	Italy	Prospective Cohort	*Fair*
5	Role of Low-Molecular-Weight Heparin in hospitalized patients with Severe Acute Respiratory Syndrome Coronavirus 2 pneumonia: A prospective observational study	Falcone M, Tiseo G, Barbieri G, Russo A, Virdis A, Forfori F, et al.	Italy	Prospective Cohort	*Good*
6	Experience with the use of baricitinib and tocilizumab monotherapy or combined, in patients with interstitial pneumonia secondary to coronavirus COVID19: A real-world study.	Rosas J, Liaño FP, Cantó ML, Barea JM, Beser AR, Rabasa JT, et al.	Spain	Case Control	*Fair*
7	Clinical outcomes in a cohort of non-ventilated COVID-19 patients with progressive hypoxemia and hyper-inflammatory response treated with baricitinib	Milligan PS, Amsden J, Norris SA, Baker RL, Myers J, Preston F, et al.	United States	Retrospective Cohort	*Fair*
8	Beneficial impact of baricitinib in COVID-19 moderate pneumonia; multicenter study.	Cantini F, Niccoli L, Nannini C, Matarrese D, Natale M Lotti P, et al.	Italy	Retrospective Cohort	*Fair*
9	Baricitinib therapy in COVID-19: A pilot study on safety and clinical impact.	Cantini F, Niccoli L, Nannini C, Matarrese D, Natale M Lotti P, et al.	Italy	Retrospective Cohort	*Fair*
10	Biological agents for rheumatic diseases in the outbreak of COVID-19: friend or foe?	Santos CS, Férnandez XC, Moriano CM, Álvarez ED, Castro CA, Robles AL, et al.	Spain	Retrospective Cohort	*Good*

S. N.	Title of study	Authors	Study location	Study design	Bias assessment
11	Baricitinib plus dexamethasone compared to dexamethasone for the treatment of severe COVID-19 pneumonia: A retrospective analysis	Pérez-Alba E, Nuzzolo-Shihadeh L, Aguirre-García G, Espinosa-Mora J, Lecona-Garcia J, Flores-Pérez R, et al.	Mexico	Retrospective Cohort	*Good*
12	The effect of baricitinib usage on the clinical and biochemical profiles of COVID-19 patients- A retrospective observational study	Amarnath A, Das A, Mutya VSS, Ibrahim I	India	Retrospective Cohort	*Fair*
13	Anakinra vs baricitinib: Different strategies for patients hospitalized with COVID-19	García-García J, Pérez-Quintana M, Ramos-Giráldez C, Cebrián-González I, Martín-Ponce M, del Valle-Villagrán J, et al	Spain	Retrospective Cohort	*Good*
14	Baricitinib improves respiratory function in patients treated with corticosteroids for SARS-CoV-2 pneumonia: an observational cohort study	Rodriguez-Garcia J, Sanchez-Nievas G, Arevalo-Serrano J, Garcia-Gomez C, Jimenez-Vizuete J, Martinez-Alfaro E.	Spain	Prospective Cohort	*Good*
15	Baricitinib against severe COVID-19: effectiveness and safety in hospitalized pretreated patients	Iglesias Gómez R, Méndez R, Palanques-Pastor T, Ballesta-López O, Borrás Almenar C, Megías Vericat J, et al.	Spain	Retrospective Cohort	*Fair*
16	Baricitinib reduces 30-day mortality in older adults with moderate-to-severe COVID-19 pneumonia	Abizanda P, Calbo Mayo J, Mas Romero M, Cortés Zamora E, Tabernero Sahuquillo M, Romero Rizos L, et al.	Spain	Retrospective Cohort	*Good*
17	Efficacy of combination therapy with the JAK inhibitor baricitinib in the treatment of COVID-19	Thomas BL, Gosselin J, Libman B, Littenberg B, Budd R C.	United States	Retrospective Cohort	*Good*
18	Combination of baricitinib plus remdesivir and dexamethasone improves time to recovery and mortality among hospitalized patients with severe COVID-19 infection (preprint)	Perez-Gutierrez V, Shah V, Afsheen A, Khalid A, Yangco A, Ocrospoma S, et al.	United States	Case Control	*Good*
19	Effect of baricitinib in patients with coronavirus disease 2019 and respiratory failure: A propensity score-matched retrospective cohort study.	Tanimoto T, Tada S, Fujita S, Hirakawa T, Matsumura M, Isoyama S, et al.	Japan	Retrospective Cohort	*Good*

S. N.	Title of study	Authors	Study location	Study design	Bias assessment
20	Efficacy of the combination of baricitinib, remdesivir, and dexamethasone in hypoxic adults with COVID-19: A retrospective study.	Yasuda Y, Hirayama Y, Uemasu K, Arasawa S, Iwashima D, Takahashi K	Japan	Retrospective Cohort	*Fair*
21	Use of baricitinib in combination with remdesivir and steroid in COVID-19 treatment: A multicenter retrospective study.	So, JM, Umeh C, Noriega S, Stratton E, Aseri M, Gupta R C	United States	Retrospective Cohort	*Good*
22	Tocilizumab, netakimab, and baricitinib in patients with mild-to-moderate COVID-19: a retrospective cohort study	Bryushkova EA, Skatova VD, Mutovina ZY, Zagrebneva AI, Fomina DS, Kruglova TS, et al.	Japan	Retrospective Cohort	*Fair*
23	Real-life effectiveness and safety of baricitinib as adjunctive to standard-of-care treatment in hospitalized patients with severe coronavirus disease 2019.	Tziolos N, Karofylakis E, Grigoropoulos I, Kazakou P, Koullias E, Savva A, et al.	Greece	Retrospective Cohort	*Good*
24	Therapeutic safety and efficacy of triple-immunosuppressants vs dual-immunosuppressants in severe-to-critical COVID-19: A prospective cohort study in Bangladesh.	Hasan MJ, Rabbani R, Anam AM, Huq SMR	Bangladesh	Prospective Cohort	*Fair*
Interventional studies					
25	Efficacy and safety of baricitinib in patients with COVID-19 infection: Results from the randomized, double-blind, placebo-controlled, parallel-group COV-BARRIER phase 3 trial.	Marconi VC, Ramanan AV, Bono S, Kartman CE, Krishnan V, Liao R, et al.	South and North America, Europe, Asia.	Double-blinded RCT	*Low*
26	Baricitinib plus remdesivir for hospitalized adults with Covid-19.	Kalil AC, Patterson TF, Mehta AK, Tomashek KM, Wolfe CR, Ghazaryan V, et al.	U.S., Singapore, South Korea, Mexico, Japan, Spain, U.K., Denmark	Double-blinded RCT	*Low*
27	Clinical impact of combination therapy with baricitinib, remdesivir, and dexamethasone in patients with severe COVID-19	Izumo T, Kuse N, Awano N, Tone M, Sakamoto K, Takada K, et al.	Japan	Double-blinded RCT	*Low*

S. N.	Title of study	Authors	Study location	Study design	Bias assessment
28	Combined administration of inhaled DNase, baricitinib and tocilizumab as rescue treatment in COVID-19 patients with severe respiratory failure	Gavriilidis E, Antoniadou C, Chrysanthopoulou A, Ntinopoulou M, Smyrlis A, Fotiadou I, et al.	Greece	Non-Randomized Open label	*Probably high risk*
29	Baricitinib plus Standard of care for hospitalized adults with COVID-19 on invasive mechanical ventilation or extracorporeal membrane oxygenation: Results of a randomized, placebo-controlled trial.	Ely EW, Ramanan AV, Cynthia EK, Bono S, Liao R, Piruzeli MLB, et al	Argentina, Brazil, Mexico, U.S.	Double-blinded RCT	*Low*
30	Baricitinib vs dexamethasone for adults hospitalized with COVID-19 (ACTT-4): A randomized, double-blind, double placebo-controlled trial	Wolfe CR, Tomashek KM, Patterson TF, Gomez CA, Marconi VC, Jain MK, et al.	United States	Double-blinded RCT	*Low*

Table 1.
Summary of the observational and interventional studies.

15 days). The NLD group required greater ICU support and mechanical ventilation (29.4% NLD vs 10% LD, $P < 0.05$ and 11.8% NLD vs 5% LD, $P = 0.141$, respectively) [24].

Titanji et al. [25] conducted a retrospective cohort study in 15 patients with moderate–severe COVID-19 pneumonia, treated with oral baricitinib (2–4 mg OD for a maximum of 7 days) and oral hydroxychloroquine (200–400 mg OD) with standard prophylactic treatment of DVT with unfractionated heparin or lower molecular weight heparin (LMWH). The combination therapy showed improved clinical status in 73% of patients in terms of fever and other presenting symptoms, oxygen requirement, and C-reactive protein (CRP) levels, with 80% survival (12/15); three patients died due to underlying pre-existing conditions. With no comparator and concurrent administration of hydroxychloroquine. With a very small study and no comparator, this study could not establish a cause-effect relationship between baricitinib treatment and outcomes.

In Verona, Italy, Bronte et al. [26] observed 76 patients with COVID-19 pneumonia prospectively, 20 of whom received 4 mg BD baricitinib for 2 days as an initial loading dose, followed by 4 mg OD for 5 days as maintenance dose, in addition to standard therapy of hydroxychloroquine and/or antivirals (ritonavir/lopinavir), along with supportive therapy with antimicrobials and anticoagulants. The mortality rate in the baricitinib cohort was significantly lower than in the standard therapy cohort [1(5%) vs 25(45%), respectively]. Similarly, the need for oxygen flow therapy was reduced ($P < 0.001$), as were serum/plasma levels of CRP ($P < 0.001$), p-STAT3 ($P < 0.001$), as well as T lymphocytes, NK cells, monocytes, IL-1, IL-6, and TNF-α concentrations in the baricitinib group. The baricitinib group also showed an absolute increase in circulating lymphocytes, IL-8 serum levels, $CD4^+$ T cells, and an increase in the PaO_2/FiO_2 ratio ($P = 0.02$). However, both cohorts faired the same with regards to acute respiratory distress syndrome (ARDS) incidence, hospitalization duration, fever resolution, lung involvement as on HR-CT/Chest X ray, $CD8^+$ T cells, the absolute number of NK (Natural Killer) cells, and expansion of monocytes.

In a prospective cohort study (with 1:1 matching) in Pisa, Italy, Falcone et al. [27] primarily evaluated the effect of LMWH treatment in 244 patients with COVID-19 pneumonia, as along with assessment of treatment effects of many drugs like hydroxychloroquine, proteases inhibitors, doxycycline, corticosteroids, macrolides, tocilizumab and remdesivir including baricitinib (n = 40 patients). Only 21 of these 40 patients, who received baricitinib along with one or more additional drugs, had matched controls and were evaluated for outcome. The univariate and multivariate regression analysis for the association between interventions and mortality revealed a hazards ratio of 0.14 (P = 0.006) and an aHR of 0.69 (P = 0.45), with a mortality of 9% with baricitinib. The hazards ratio for death/severe ARDS was 0.53 (P = 0.12). When baricitinib intervention was matched with mortality and severe ARDS, and regression analysis was performed, the HRs were 1.35 (0.32–5.96) and 1.38 (0.48–4.01), respectively, with P values of 0.678 and 0.54. The study found no significant beneficial (or harmful) effect of baricitinib on the clinical recovery of COVID-19 pneumonia patients, but it was clearly underpowered to evaluate the effect of baricitinib.

In a retrospective observational study, Rosas et al. [28] compared the effect of baricitinib and tocilizumab as monotherapies or in combination with the standard of care therapy used for COVID-19 in Spain among 60 patients. The baricitinib group (n = 12) received 2 or 4 mg orally, tocilizumab group (n = 20) received weight adjusted dose of 400–600 mg, combination group (n = 11) received both baricitinib and tocilizumab and a fourth group (n = 17) received neither of the therapies. The patients received drugs such as antivirals, azithromycin, hydroxychloroquine, interferon, corticosteroid apart from the above therapies. More than 50% of patients were over the age of 70 years. The study revealed no significant mortality benefits of either of the treatment regimens. When compared to the standard of care group (neither tocilizumab or baricitinib), the baricitinib monotherapy group showed a significant reduction in temperature, CRP, D-Dimer, oxygen saturation, and respiratory rate ($P < 0.05$), and the combination group (tocilizumab + baricitinib) showed a similar but more significant difference ($P < 0.01$). When baricitinib was compared to tocilizumab monotherapy, it showed greater reductions in CRP, D-Dimer, respiratory rate, lymphocytosis, LDH, and temperature. During the study, no relevant side effects were recorded with either of the therapies. Baseline comparison revealed that the patients receiving baricitinib/tocilizumab presented with a more serious (worsened) disease in comparison to those who received neither drug.

Milligan et al. [29] conducted a retrospective longitudinal study in 22 patients with COVID-19 pneumonia and compared the effect of baricitinib (2 mg OD orally for 7 days) to the standard of care (hydroxychloroquine ± ribavirin ± corticosteroids and anticoagulant treatment). The baseline characteristics of the participants differed significantly. The study found clinical improvement in patients receiving baricitinib therapy; 16 patients did not experience disease progression, while the remaining patients died (n = 3) or required mechanical ventilation. Prior to the completion of the baricitinib regimen, the oxygen demands of the majority of the patients (77.3%) improved by at least one WHO oxygenation criteria. Ferritin and CRP levels fell significantly from a median of 885 to 326.5 ng/ml and 20.35 ng/ml to 17.3 mg/dl, respectively. Baricitinib caused mild adverse effects such as thrombocytosis (n = 22), transaminase elevation (n = 5), while acute kidney injury, AKI (n = 2), lymphopenia (n = 1) led to treatment discontinuations.

Cantini et al. [15] conducted a pilot ambivalent cohort study in Italy, enrolling 12 patients with moderate COVID-19 who received baricitinib in addition to standard antiviral and hydroxychloroquine therapy. Another 12 patients were matched from previous hospital records to serve as controls, who had received the then-standard of care therapy. Overall, clinical characteristics and respiratory function parameters improved significantly in the baricitinib-treated group. CRP levels decreased significantly after 14 days, whereas no significant changes were observed in the controls. While none of the baricitinib-treated patients requested ICU transfer, 33% (4/12) of the controls did ($P = 0.093$). In comparison to 8% (1/12) of the controls, 58% (7/12) of the baricitinib-treated patients were discharged at 14 days ($P = 0.027$). Fever, SpO_2, PaO_2/FiO_2, CRP, and the Modified Early Warning Score (MEWS) all improved significantly when compared to controls.

The same team of researchers also conducted a retrospective longitudinal multicentric study in patients who had previously been hospitalized with moderate COVID-19 to compare the effectiveness of standard therapy ($n = 78$) and baricitinib ($n = 113$) administered over the course of 2 weeks as an add-on to lopinavir/ritonavir and LMWH. The 2-week case-fatality rate was found to be significantly lower in the baricitinib group as compared to the control group (0 vs 6.4% in baricitinib vs control, $P = 0.01$), along with lesser ICU admissions (0.88 vs 17.9%). SpO_2, PaO_2/FiO_2, transaminase levels, and lymphocyte counts were significantly increased in the baricitinib group, while CRP and IL-6 levels were significantly decreased. At discharge, the baricitinib group had a significantly lower proportion of patients who tested positive for COVID-19 on pharyngeal swabs (2.5 vs 40% in controls) [16].

Santol et al. [30] studied the incidence of COVID-19 pneumonia in patients receiving disease-modifying anti-rheumatic drugs (DMARDs) retrospectively. COVID was contracted by 40 of 820 rheumatic disease patients. Among the three patients were being treated with baricitinib, none developed COVID, indicating that the drug may have a protective effect. The study's major limitations were the very low number of COVID-19 cases and patients receiving baricitinib.

In a Mexican retrospective cohort study [31], Alba et al. compared baricitinib in combination with dexamethasone ($n = 123$) to dexamethasone alone ($n = 74$) among hospitalized patients with severe COVID-19. Overall 30-day mortality was significantly lower in the combination therapy group (20.3%) than in the dexamethasone monotherapy group (40.5%); $P < 0.05$. Combination therapy did not increase the risk of hospital acquired infections.

Another retrospective study from India [32] described the clinical and biochemical parameters of 31 patients with moderate-to-severe COVID-19 who were treated with a combination of baricitinib and remdesivir. At baseline, over 50% of patients were males, diabetic, had at least one comorbidity, and all of them received steroids along with baricitinib and remdesivir. The treatment reduced oxygen requirement over the course of hospitalization ($P < 0.05$), reduced CRP levels from an average of 93.9 to 32.3 ($P = 0.0001$), IL-6 values from an average of 47.5 to 20.8 ($P = 0.004$), and the neutrophil lymphocyte ratio (NLR), with no significant changes in ferritin or D-dimer. The study also performed a subgroup analysis, which showed that oxygen requirement was higher in older age groups, reduced in individuals with comorbidities, absent in those with no comorbidities, and showed a decrease in all survivors. The CRP value, IL-6, NLR, D-dimer and ferritin all showed a similar trend of reduction with treatment in older age groups and comorbidities.

Garcia-Garcia et al. [33] carried out a retrospective cohort study in Spain to compare the effect of IL-1 inhibitor anakinra ($n = 125$) vs baricitinib ($n = 217$) as an add-on to corticosteroid and standard care therapy in hospitalized patients with COVID-19 pneumonia, and found no differences in mortality (17.6 vs 16.6%). However, a significantly lower proportion of patients receiving baricitinib required invasive mechanical ventilation than those receiving anakinra (4.6 vs 10.4%; $P = 0.039$).

Garcia-Rodriguez et al. [34] in a prospective cohort study, compared improvement in pulmonary function in patients with moderate to severe COVID-19 pneumonia treated with corticosteroids ($n = 50$) vs combination of corticosteroids and baricitinib ($n = 62$), both in addition to lopinavir/ritonavir and hydroxychloroquine. The combination group improved SpO_2/FiO_2 significantly more than the corticosteroid alone group (mean difference 49; 95% CI 22–77, $P < 0.001$). Similarly, a significantly lower proportion of patients in the combination group required supplemental oxygen at discharge and 1 month (25.8%, 12.9%) compared to those in the corticosteroid alone group (62%, 28%), with ORs of 0.18 and 0.31 respectively.

In a retrospective analysis by Gómez et al. in Spain [35], 43 hospitalized severe COVID-19 patients ($SpO_2 < 92\%$) received barictinib 4 mg orally for 5–7 days; Majority (84%) of these patients were additionally administered corticosteroids. On an 8-category ordinal scale, a substantial median clinical improvement of 3 points (IQR 1–4) was noted from day 1 to day 15 ($P < 0.01$). There was no mortality by days 30 and 60, and all participants were discharged with clinical improvement. The median recovery time was 12 days. All clinical measures associated with poor prognosis in COVID-19 showed a substantial improvement ($P < 0.05$), and no noteworthy adverse effects were reported.

In a retrospective cohort study, Abizanda et al. [36] enrolled 328 older adults with moderate to severe COVID-19 pneumonia ($n = 164$ each on baricitinib and propensity score matched controls). They were divided into two groups: <70 years old ($n = 86$) and ≥70 years old ($n = 78$), receiving a mean total dose of 17.6 ± 10.2 mg baricitinib for a mean 5.9 days of treatment. A few participants were also given tocilizumab, anakinra, and corticosteroids. When using Cox proportional hazard models adjusted for important covariates, patients in the ≥70 age group had a significantly lower 30-day fatality rate with baricitinib (HR 0.21; 95% CI 0.09–0.47; $P < 0.001$). Despite a higher disease severity in the baricitinib group, similar results were found in those <70 (HR 0.14; 95% CI 0.03–0.64; $P = 0.011$). This study demonstrated baricitinib's clinical utility and safety in the important subset of elderly patients.

Thoms et al. [37], in their retrospective longitudinal study in the U.S., observed the impact of short course baricitinib therapy (4 mg daily either as single dose or two divided doses) in 45 COVID-19 positive in-patients in addition to IV remdesivir with a loading dose of 200 mg and 100 mg maintenance dose for 4 days along with dexamethasone 6 mg IV for 10 days. The patients had an average age of 65 years with a predominance of female gender. The average treatment duration was 6 days. Results showed a 4.4% mortality over the first 7 days of admission and 13.3% over the entire duration of hospitalization among patients, with oxygen supplementation in some format required for all participants. There was a reversal in the downward trend of hemoglobin levels post commencement of treatment along with CRP, D-dimer, and ferritin, and along with increased platelet counts. The Adaptive COVID-19 Treatment Trial—Clinical Status (ACTT-CS) scores also showed a significant statistical improvement in response to therapy. Four patients were reported to have experienced a hemodynamic shock requiring a vasopressor.

Gutierrez et al. [38] conducted a case control study in New York city consisting of 139 COVID patients, and compared the effect of dexamethasone 6 mg OD with remdesivir 200 mg IV followed by 100 mg daily IV for 10 days (Standard of Care,

SOC) and a combination of baricitinib 4 mg OD with remdesivir for 10 days. The SOC group consisted of 51 individuals serving as controls, and 88 patients who received SOC plus baricitinib were considered as cases. The groups displayed similar baseline characteristics. Thirty-three patients received mechanical ventilation overall, of which 14 were in standard therapy (27.45%) and 19 (21.59%) in the baricitinib group. There was an increased need for antibiotics in the controls over the cases (76.5 vs 53.4%, $P = 0.007$). The individuals who received baricitinib displayed a reduction in median time to recovery by 3 days compared to the control group, but this difference was not statistically significant. The study also performed stratification based on oxygen requirement, and those with low flow oxygen (OS5) and high flow nasal cannula (OS6) both showed significant reductions in median time to recovery (OS 5: 3 days lesser, rate ratio of recovery of 2.95 in 95% CI, 1.03–8.42, $P = 0.04$, OS 6: 2 days lesser, Rate Ratio 1.80, 95% CI, 1.09–2.98, $P = 0.02$).

Tanimoto et al. [39], in their propensity score-matched retrospective cohort study, recruited 229 patients in Hiroshima, Japan, to study the effect of baricitinib in comparison to standard of care on 30 and 60 day survival after admission. Other drugs such as favipiravir, corticosteroids, remdesivir, heparin and tocilizumab were also administered to both groups in similar proportions. A logistic regression model was used to designate two propensity matched cohorts of similar age, sex, severity of disease, BMI, comorbidities, and usage of other drugs. The 30-day survival was significantly higher in the baricitinib propensity score-matched cohort ($P = 0.03$) whereas there was no significant statistical difference in the 60-day survival. Other outcomes of significance were the need for oxygen therapy in the cohorts where a smaller proportion of individuals in the baricitinib group required oxygen ($P < 0.001$), and a better outcome at discharge in the baricitinib cohort ($P = 0.02$). There were no significant differences in the adverse events reported in either group.

Yasuda et al. [40] carried out a single centre retrospective study in Osaka, Japan, where they recruited 108 COVID-19 positive patients. Of them, 16 were treated with dexamethasone only (6 mg daily for 10 days), 2 with standard of care, 30 received the combination of 3 drugs (baricitinib 4 mg or 2 mg for 2 weeks or until no more requirement of oxygen therapy with dexamethasone and remdesivir IV with a loading dose of 200 mg and maintenance dose of 100 mg for 5 days), and 60 with only remdesivir and dexamethasone (controls). At baseline, the baricitinib group had significantly younger individuals ($P = 0.006$), as well as significantly more severe chest X ray abnormalities ($P = 0.0248$). Patients in the baricitinib group experienced a faster recovery (3 days less, $P < 0.001$), with a recovery rate of 90% in the baricitinib group and 63.3% in the control group ($P = 0.011$). All-cause mortality was also significantly lower in baricitinib (6.7 vs 28.3%, $P = 0.0263$), with a ratio of recovery at 5.26 (95% CI, 1.99–13.9, $P < 0.001$). Among the 39 patients receiving oral anticoagulants, the recovery rate was 90 vs 44.4% (baricitinib vs control, $P = 0.0089$). The study identified age and anticoagulants to be significantly associated with recovery time. Baricitinib showed an accelerated recovery in patients aged 65 years or above ($P = 0.039$) but no such difference in those below 65 years of age ($P = 0.307$).

So et al. [41], in their retrospective cohort study, included 100 COVID-19 diagnosed patients in Southern California, U.S., to compare the efficacy of baricitinib in comparison to other treatment regimens used in the hospital. Those who received baricitinib were *less likely* to be in the intensive care units as compared to those who did not (45.8% of ICU patients took baricitinib and 56.2% did not, $P = 0.017$). Kaplan–Meier analysis revealed that patients who received baricitinib have an increased survival as compared to those who did not (26 days, 95% CI 11.7–40.3, vs

14 days, 95% CI 12.4–15.6, $P = 0.045$). The study also revealed that 33% of patients on baricitinib showed an elevation of liver enzymes post commencement of drug administration but not severe enough to indicate an abrupt discontinuation of treatment and returned to normal after stopping treatment.

Bryushkova et al. [42], in their retrospective cohort study on 154 COVID-19 patients in Moscow, Russia, compared the effects of three drugs namely baricitinib, netakimab and tocilizumab along with the standard of care including hydroxychloroquine (400 mg BD on day 1 and 200 mg BD on days 5–10), azithromycin (500 mg once per day for 5 days), lopinavir–ritonavir (400/100 mg twice per day for 14 days), and low molecular-weight heparin according to indications. The cohorts consisted of 38 individuals who received baricitinib, 48 received netakimab, 34 received tocilizumab and 34 received only the standard of care, and showed significant baseline differences in neutrophil lymphocyte ratio, lactate dehydrogenase (LDH) and NEWS-2 median score among the cohorts. The CRP and LDH levels showed significant reduction in the tocilizumab group and netakimab group but not in baricitinib and SOC after 72 h; reduced in all groups majorly after 120 h. In similar trends, NEWS-2 score improved in 72 h for tocilizumab and netakimab, and in 120 h for tocilizumab, netakimab and baricitinib. The NLR showed a decrease in the baricitinib group but an improvement in netakimab and tocilizumab groups. In comparison to the baricitinib (31.6%) and SOC (23.5%) groups, the proportion of patients who were discharged 5–7 days after the initiation of therapy was greater in the tocilizumab (44.1%) and netakimab (41.7%) groups. The SOC (9%) and baricitinib (3%) groups had greater mortality rates than tocilizumab (0%) and netakimab (0%) groups.

A retrospective cohort study conducted by Tziolos et al. [43] in Athens, Greece assessed the role of baricitinib (4 mg/day for 14 days or discharge) as an add-on therapy to the standard of care in 369 hospitalized patients with COVID-19 which included dexamethasone (6 mg/day), remdesivir (200 mg/day on day 1 followed by 100 mg/day for subsequent days) and low molecular weight heparin for thromboprophylaxis apart from antimicrobials as per the physicians discretion. The standard of care regimen was provided to 47.7% of the patients and the remaining received baricitinib as an add-on. At baseline, patients in the standard of care group showed increase comorbidities of hypertension, CVD, heart failure, end stage renal disease (ESRD) and active neoplastic or inflammatory disease and those in the baricitinib group were significantly younger (61.6 ± 12.7 vs 69.1 ± 13.5 years, $P < 0.001$), received remdesivir more often, and an intermediate dose of LMWH and oxygen by high flow nasal cannula ($P < 0.05$ for both). The baricitinib combination showed a reduced overall mortality (14.7 vs 26.6%, $P = 0.005$), achieved a lower composite outcome of ICU admission and all-cause mortality (22.3 vs 36.9%, $P = 0.002$). When subgroup analysis as per ARDS severity was performed, the mortality, and the composite outcome was statistically significant in favor of the combination group for both subgroups. No significant difference in thromboembolic events were seen in either group.

Hasan et al. [44], in their third published study on use of baricitinib in COVID-19, conducted a prospective cohort study in 103 adult patients who were divided into two groups by simple random sampling as 49 participants in group A (receiving baricitinib 4 mg OD PO for 14 days plus secukinumab two doses 48 h apart 300 mg IV) and 54 participants in group B (baricitinib plus secukinumab single dose in similar doses as A plus tocilizumab 8 mg/Kg single dose IV). All patients received dexamethasone 0.25 mg/Kg in divided doses, remdesivir 200 mg IV loading plus 100 mg maintenance for 10 days IV, LMWH, and antimicrobials for infections. The number of male patients in both groups was higher and the median time of hospitalization was 7 and 9 days in group A and B respectively. Group B showed a quicker median day to achieve normal SpO_2, lower requirement of ICU and mechanical ventilation (N = 54) 28.6%/16.7% (P = 004); 18.4%/11.1% (P = 038), lower risk of ARDS (OR = 0.43, P = 0.045) and a lower 60 day all-cause mortality 14.29% (N 1/4 49) vs 7.41% (N 1/4 54); OR 0.35 (0.08–1.44), 95% CI). However, group B also showed a higher rate of adverse events.

2.2 Interventional studies

Marconi et al. [45] published the findings of the phase 3 COV BARRIER trial, a randomized placebo-controlled double blind study that enrolled adult hospitalized symptomatic COVID-19 patients who required low flow oxygen and had atleast one elevated inflammatory marker (CRP, D-dimer, LDH, ferritin). This trial was carried out at 101 sites in 12 countries across South and North America, Europe, and Asia. It enrolled a total of 1525 participants who received either oral baricitinib 4 mg (n = 764) or placebo once daily for 14 days (1:1), in addition to standard of care (SOC), which included low dose systemic corticosteroids (79.3%, mostly dexamethasone), remdesivir (18.9%), and anticoagulants. All patients were monitored for disease progression and mortality until day 28 and then again until day 60. No significant difference was seen in the proportion of patients who progressed (requiring high flow oxygen, non-invasive/invasive ventilation, or death) after treatment with baricitinib vs placebo [27.8 vs 30.5%; OR 0.85, 95% CI 0.67–1.08; P = 0.18] on day 28. However, in a prespecified secondary endpoint analysis, baricitinib significantly reduced the all-cause mortality on day 28 compared to placebo (8.1 vs 13.1%, HR 0.57, 95% CI 0.41–0.78, P = 0.0018). On day 60 also, mortality was reduced significantly (HR 0.62, 95% CI 0.47–0.83, P = 0.005). The survival benefits were more pronounced in patients with more severe disease at baseline. There were no appreciable differences in treatment-emergent adverse events (44.5 vs 44.4%), serious adverse events (14.7 vs 18%), serious infections, or venous thromboembolic events between baricitinib vs placebo. The trial showed that the combination of baricitinib and corticosteroid therapy significantly lowers mortality among patients of moderate—severe COVID-19 who are hospitalized.

The results of the first stage of the Adaptive COVID-19 Treatment Trial (ACTT-1) demonstrating the efficacy of remdesivir treatment in hospitalized COVID-19 patients with pneumonia were released in May 2020 [46]. In ACTT-2 [47], the efficacy of treatment with remdesivir in combination with baricitinib was compared to remdesivir plus placebo (control) in 1033 hospitalized adults with COVID-19. The combination group patients (n = 515) were given oral baricitinib at a daily dose of 4 mg for 14 days, or until hospital discharge/death along with IV remdesivir in a loading dose of 200 mg on day one, followed by a maintenance dose of 100 mg from day 2 to day 10, or until hospital discharge/death Patients who got remdesivir in combination with baricitinib had quicker recovery than those who received only remdesivir (median 7 vs 8 days; RR for recovery 1.16; 95% CI 1.01–1.32; P = 0.03). The combination group had a faster median time to recovery of 10 days compared to 18 days among patients getting high flow oxygen or non-invasive ventilation (RR 1.51; 95% CI 1.10–2.08). The RR of recovery was 0.88 (95% CI 0.63–1.23), 1.17 (95% CI 0.98–1.39) and 1.08 (95% CI 0.59–1.97) for patients who received no oxygen, supplemental oxygen, and mechanical ventilation respectively. After 28 days, the overall mortality rate was relatively lower in the combination group (5.1 vs 7.8%, HR 0.65;

95% CI 0.39–1.09). Patients who received supplemental oxygen had a relatively lower mortality rate than those who received high flow oxygen (1.9 vs 4.7%; HR 0.40; 95% CI 0.14–1.14 or non-invasive ventilation (7.5 vs 12.9%; HR 0.55; 95% CI 0.22–1.38), but results were not statistically significant. Patients in the combination group recovered in 6 days on an average compared to 8 days in the control group (RR 1.21; 95% CI 1.06–1.39). In the combination group, 40.7% (n = 207) patients experienced grade 3 or 4 adverse events (anemia, hyperglycemia, decreased lymphocyte count, and acute kidney injury), compared to 46.8% (n = 238) patients in the remdesivir group. Among these, a significantly higher proportion of patients experienced serious adverse events in the remdesivir group (21%) compared to the combination group (16%); a difference of −5.0% (95% CI, −9.8 to −0.3; P = 0.03). This trial concluded that baricitinib in combination with remdesivir is superior and safer than remdesivir alone, with fewer serious adverse events. Combination therapy also helps patients recover faster and accelerates improvements in clinical status, especially among those who require high flow oxygen or non-invasive ventilation.

A small interventional study was conducted by Izumo et al. [48] in Tokyo, Japan, on COVID-19 patients with severe or critical disease without renal dysfunction. A total of 44 patients were given a triple combination therapy of oral baricitinib 4 mg (up to 14 days), standard IV remdesivir regimen (up to 10 days), and IV dexamethasone 6 mg (up to 10 days). Overall, the results demonstrated that mortality was low (2.3%), with no need for invasive mechanical breathing in majority of patients (90%). The median length of hospitalization was 11 days whereas ICU stay was 6 days on an average, with a 9-day median recovery time. Adverse events were reported in 34% (15/44) patients. This was the first trial to demonstrate the safety and efficacy of a triple combination of baricitinib, remdesivir and corticosteroids in hospitalized COVID-19 patients. However, its primary weakness was the lack of a comparison group.

Through a non-randomized open label study in Greece, Gavriilidis et al. [49] analyzed the effect of various treatment modalities in the reduction of in-hospital mortality in 78 RT-PCR diagnosed COVID-19 patients. Participants were categorized into four groups: 26 patients received standard of Care (SOC) that included dexamethasone 6–8 mg OD, LMWH, antibiotic prophylaxis and supportive care, 11 patients received SOC and tocilizumab intravenously at a single dose of 8 mg/kg body weight (TOCI), 19 patients received SOC plus anakinra at a dosage of 200 mg BD for 3–6 days followed by 100 mg BD up to 10 days (ANA) and the COMBI group of 22 patients received a combination of tocilizumab, anakinra, dornase alfa (2500 IU/BD for 2 weeks) with budesonide (800 ug/BD) and salbutamol, and baricitinib at 4 mg OD if GFR >60 ml/min or 2 mg OD for 2 weeks. The baseline characteristics of all groups were similar. The SOC group observed 9 deaths (34.6%) and 10 intubations (38.5%) with a mean duration of hospital stay of 19.4 days, the ANA group had 6 deaths and intubations (31.6%) with an average duration of hospital stay of 23.9 days, the TOCI group showed 7 deaths (63.6%) and an average duration of 19.4 days of hospital stay and the COMBI group showed the lowest mortality of 2 deaths (9.1%, P = 0.014), lowest intubation rate (P = 0.013) and the lowest average hospital stay of 15.6 days (P = 0.019). Apart from these outcomes, the COMBI group also showed a prolonged survival (P = 0.003) after a median follow up of 110 days, an increase in ALC count (P = 0.021), and reduction in CRP levels (P = 0.002). Though the study demonstrates a reduction in mortality with the combination therapy including baricitinib, the lack of randomization and unequal group sizes are important limitations.

Wesley et al. [50] have published the results of an exploratory trial following the phase 3 COV-BARRIER trial which was a multicentric (18 centers across Argentina, Brazil, Mexico and the U.S.A.), randomized, double-blinded placebo controlled parallel group trial to compare the effect of baricitinib on all-cause mortality at day 28 and 60, overall improvement of clinical status, duration of hospitalization or time to recovery in COVID-19 patients. This study recruited 101 participants randomized 1:1 into baricitinib 4 mg or 2 mg if GFR < 60, l/min/1.73 m^2 (n = 51) and placebo (n = 50) for 14 days or up to discharge. All participants received the standard of care which included medications such as corticosteroids, antivirals, vasopressors, and prophylaxis for venous thromboembolic events as per local practice. All participants had at least one underlying comorbid condition. The median duration of treatment exposure was 12 days in the placebo group and 11 in the baricitinib group. The baricitinib group significantly reduced all-cause mortality by day 28 (39% in baricitinib vs 58% in placebo, HR 0.54, 95% CI 0.31–0.94., P = 0.03) with a 46% relative reduction and 19% absolute risk reduction, with a similar significant reduction at day 60 also (23 [45%] events vs 31 [62%]; HR 0.56 [95% CI 0.33–0.97]; P = 0.027; 44% relative reduction; absolute risk reduction 17%). The study revealed no significant differences in the number of ventilator free days or mean duration of hospitalization. Both groups showed a high proportion of treatment-emergent adverse events where 44 of 50 participants (88%) in the baricitinib group and 47 out of 49 (96%) in the placebo group reported at least one event, while 50% in the baricitinib arm and 71% of the placebo arm reported at least one serious adverse event, causing 28 and 35% of the patients to discontinue treatment in the baricitinib and placebo group respectively. There were five (10%) and three (6%) deaths due to adverse events in the baricitinib and placebo arm respectively. Overall, the study supported the results of the COV BARRIER trial by showing consistent results in reducing mortality in critically ill hospitalized patients with COVID-19 for baricitinib compared with placebo (plus standard of care, including corticosteroids), albeit in a small sample size.

Most recently, the results of ACTT-4 have been published (May 2022) [51], in which 1010 hospitalized patients with COVID-19 requiring supplemental oxygen or non-invasive mechanical ventilation were randomized to receive either baricitinib plus remdesivir (51%, n = 503) or dexamethasone plus remdesivir (49%, n = 482) at 67 sites across the world. All patients received remdesivir (≤10 days) and either baricitinib for a maximum of 14 days or dexamethasone for a maximum of 10 days. There was no difference between the two groups in the primary outcome of mechanical ventilation-free survival by day 29 [87.0% in the baricitinib plus remdesivir vs 87.6% in the dexamethasone plus remdesivir group; risk difference 0.6 (95% CI −3.6 to 4.8 and P = 0.91)]. Similar results were seen with odds ratio for improved clinical status at day 15 which was similar between the two groups. Outcomes were statistically similar for mortality at 29 days (2.9 vs 4.7% for baricitinib vs dexamethasone combination groups) or 60 days (6.8 vs 8%). Outcomes were consistently similar among different geographical regions, gender, race, and ethnicity as well. The safety analysis showed that 4% of patients in the baricitinib plus remdesivir group and 10% of patients in the dexamethasone plus remdesivir group experienced at least one treatment-related adverse event (risk difference: 60%; P = 000041). So, when combined with remdesivir, baricitinib is a significantly safer treatment option than dexamethasone, with severe or life-threatening grade 3 or 4 adverse events occurring in 28% of patients in the baricitinib plus remdesivir group compared to 36% of patients in the dexamethasone plus remdesivir group (P = 0012).

3. Summary of evidence

The COVID-19 pandemic has presented extremely challenging conditions for clinicians across the globe due to its infectivity, morbidity and mortality, characterized by the spread of lethal pneumonia in up to 15–20% of the cases [11]. The current therapeutic strategies for hospitalized patients are focused on the use of anti-inflammatory agents like corticosteroids, IL-6 inhibitors, antivirals agents like remdesivir, molnupiravir or a few monoclonal antibodies in combination with standard supportive care. There is still a need for more therapeutic alternatives for the hospitalized COVID-19 patients who are at risk of developing life-threatening complications such as ARDS and multiorgan dysfunction. In this context, the US FDA granted a EUA in November 2020 for baricitinib, an oral Janus Kinase inhibitor that inhibits cytokine release, to be used at a dose of 4 mg once daily in hospitalized adult patients with moderate to severe COVID-19 pneumonia in combination with remdesivir.. The FDA revised this EUA in July 2021 to allow the use of baricitinib alone (without remdesivir) for the treatment of COVID-19 in hospitalized adults and children ≥2 years of age who require supplemental oxygen, non-invasive or invasive mechanical ventilation, or ECMO [6]. Finally, in May 2022, the FDA has given full approval to baricitinib to be used for hospitalized COVID-19 adult patients as per the same conditions laid out in the EUA, while the use in children is still under the EUA.

In this chapter, we have attempted to meticulously unearth the evidence regarding the use of baricitinib as an anti-inflammatory drug for the treatment of COVID-19. Data from published observational and interventional studies reveal promising immunomodulatory and anti-inflammatory effects of baricitinib as monotherapy or in combination with other drugs in improving clinical and biochemical parameters, and other relevant disease markers in patients hospitalized with moderate to severe COVID-19. A lot of the initial evidence has come from observational studies on different drugs being tried in patients admitted in hospitals due to COVID-19, rather than the conventional gold standard RCTs; the published observational studies of different types outnumber the published interventional trials. Though the quality of evidence from observational studies (or NRSIs) may be relatively lower, the sheer number of parallel conclusions, supported by the evidence from the limited RCTs point to substantial benefits of using baricitinib in the treatment of COVID-19.

Among the multiple studies attempted to investigate clinical benefits of baricitinib in hospitalized COVID patients, some have compared the efficacy of baricitinib alone to the standard of care (antivirals, immunomodulators, protease inhibitors etc.), with different dosing regimens or loading dosages, and others have studied baricitinib as a part of a multi-drug pharmacological treatment regimens with different comparators. Despite the considerable heterogeneity in terms of study populations, sites, study designs, treatment regimens, significant study limitations, as well as the differences in summary measures, the evidence available is largely in favor of utility of the drug in COVID-19 in improving key clinical outcomes and/or biochemical or laboratory parameters, supported by an acceptable/satisfactory safety profile.

Among the 24 observational studies which include 16 retrospective cohort, 5 prospective cohort, and 3 case control studies, baricitinib has been compared to other drugs such as tocilizumab [28], used in various doses [23, 34], and therapeutic effects of loading dose changes or combination with other drugs have been assessed [24–29, 34] including IL-6 inhibitors, steroids and LMWHs like enoxaparin. The majority of the findings favor baricitinib due to its benefits in improving COVID-19 in terms of clinical, biochemical, and other disease characteristics. However, baricitinib treatment did not result in a substantial reduction in mortality in some of the studies [24, 27, 28]. Few studies also revealed an increased incidence of adverse reactions such as mouth sores [23], infections [29], and thrombocytopenia [23, 28] with baricitinib treatment. But no study showed an inferiority of baricitinib in efficacy. Major drawbacks stem from the observational nature which introduces numerous methodological limitations and flaws along with biases, and the short duration of treatment and/or follow up periods along with limited sample sizes. Key concerns in these studies include selection bias and confounding errors resulting from lack of randomization which were addressed to some extent in few studies; most could not.. Among the observational studies, 11 received a "fair" score and 13 received a "good" score when evaluated using the study quality evaluation tool [22], validated for evaluating observational research quality.

The findings of three large randomized controlled trials (RCTs) have been published. ACTT-2 results led to the EUA for baricitinib (with remdesivir) in hospitalized COVID-19 patients. The trial found that baricitinib + remdesivir (and standard of care) significantly reduced median time of recovery and mortality rate compared to control group (5.1 vs 7.8%) [47]. A similar reduction in mortality by 38.2% was also reported by Marconi et al.. in the experimental arm of oral baricitinib 4 mg plus standard treatment compared to controls who received placebo in addition to standard treatment (34). There was also improvement in participants' requirement for oxygen therapy especially in those who received high flow oxygen or for non-invasive ventilation. Encouragingly, fewer episodes of severe adverse events were seen in participants belonging to the baricitinib group compared to the standard of care. The ACTT-4 trial compared the combination of remdesivir with baricitinib or dexamethasone in hospitalized patients with COVID-19 requiring supplemental oxygen or non-invasive ventilation and showed that both combinations resulted in similar efficacy outcomes like mechanical ventilation-free survival by day 29, mortality and clinical status improvement. However, the baricitinib combination was found to be safer as dexamethasone was associated with significantly higher proportion of treatment-related adverse events, as well as severe or life-threatening adverse events [51]. The risk of bias was assessed using the risk of bias (ROB 2.0) tool [21]. All three RCTs were graded as having overall 'low risk of bias'. Besides these RCTs, results of three other interventional trials also support similar findings for the clinical utility of baricitinib among different COVID-19 patient populations.

As results from more ongoing RCTs get published, the evidence is likely to grow stronger.

3.1 Ongoing clinical trials

In addition to the published data, it is important to review the key ongoing registered clinical trials on use of baricitinib in treatment of COVID-19 to gain an understanding of the type of evidence expected in the future. There are currently multiple (>10) ongoing clinical trials evaluating the safety and efficacy of oral baricitinib alone or in combination for treatment of COVID-19 patients. **Table 2** provides key features of some of these registered trials, usually multicentric RCTs, listed on global clinical trial registries whose results have not been declared or published. One trial each is in phase III and IV, one is in phase II/III, four are in phase II, and one is in phase Ib/II.

Among the late phase trials, the TACTIC-R is a phase IV multi-arm platform trial proposed to be conducted at multiple centers across U.K. [52, 61]. It is a parallel 3-arm

S. N.	Trial identifierand phase	Trial setting - Patient population	Last updated status	Official title	Sponsor/lead institution, Country
1	NCT-04390464 [52] Phase- IV	Hospitalized	Recruiting status unknown	mulTi-Arm Therapeutic study in pre-ICu patients admitted with Covid-19—Repurposed Drugs (TACTIC-R):	Cambridge University Hospitals NHS Foundation Trust United Kingdom
2	NCT-04832880 [53, 54] Phase- III	Hospitalized	Not yet recruiting	Factorial, Multicentric, Randomized Clinical Trial of Remdesivir and Immunotherapy in Combination with Dexamethasone for Moderate COVID-19 (the AMMURAVID Trial)	ASST Fatebenefratelli Sacco Italy
3	NCT-04320277 [55] Phase- II/III	Hospitalized	Recruiting status unknown	Baricitinib Combined with Antiviral Therapy in Symptomatic Patients Infected by COVID-19: an Open-label, Pilot Study (BARI-COVID)	Hospital of Prato Italy
4	NCT-04399798 [56] Phase- II	Hospitalized	Recruiting status unknown	Baricitinib for coRona Virus pnEumonia (COVID-19): a THerapeutic Trial (BREATH): A proof-of Concept Study of the Use of Janus Kinase 1 and 2 Inhibitor, Baricitinib, in the Treatment of COVID-19-related Pneumonia:	IRCCS Policlinico S. Matteo Italy
5	NCT-04393051 [57] Phase- II	Hospitalized	Recruiting status unknown	BARICIVID-19 STUDY: Multicenter, Randomized, Phase IIa Clinical Trial Evaluating Efficacy and Tolerability of Baricitinib as add-on Treatment of In-patients With COVID-19 Compared to Standard Therapy	Azienda Ospedaliero, Universitaria Pisana Italy
6	NCT-04346147 [58] Phase- II	Hospitalized	Active, not recruiting	Clinical Trial to Evaluate Efficacy of 3 Types of Treatment in Patients with Pneumonia by COVID-19 (Covid19COVINIB): Prospective, Phase II, Randomized, Open-label, Parallel Group Study to Evaluate the Efficacy of Baricitinib, Imatinib or Supportive Treatment in Patients with SARS Cov2 Pneumonia	Hospital Universitario de Fuenlabrada Spain

S. N.	Trial identifierand phase	Trial setting - Patient population	Last updated status	Official title	Sponsor/lead institution, Country
7	NCT-04321993 [59] Phase- II	Hospitalized	Recruiting	Treatment of Moderate to Severe Coronavirus Disease (COVID-19) in Hospitalized Patients	Lisa Barrett, Nova Scotia Health Authority Canada
8	20-0356 [60] Phase- Ib/II	Hospitalized	Recruiting	A Phase I/II Clinical Trial to evaluate the efficacy of baricitinib to prevent respiratory insufficiency progression in onco-hematological patients affected with COVID19: A structured summary of a study protocol for a randomized controlled trial	Institutional Crowd Funding Spain

Table 2.
Registered on-going clinical trials to evaluate the efficacy and safety of baricitinib in COVID-19 patients.

(1:1:1) randomized trial evaluating baricitinib 4 mg OD and ravulizumab as a potential treatment for COVID-19 among hospitalized patients in comparison to standard treatment alone over a 14-day treatment period with follow-ups at day 28 and day 90 post-discharge. The safety and efficacy of different treatment arms will be assessed on a 7-point pulmonary scale, death, invasive mechanical ventilation, non-invasive ventilation or high flow oxygen, low flow oxygen, no oxygen, and status at discharge.

The phase III AMMURAVID RCT is proposed to be conducted across 21 study locations in Italy [53, 54] and is expected to enroll approximately 4000 participants with hospitalized COVID-19. The trial aims at evaluating the efficacy of remdesivir, baricitinib (4 mg), and remdesivir plus baricitinib vs the control arm (IV dexamethasone 6 mg × 10 days). The primary objective is minimization of progression of severe respiratory failure in COVID-19, as well as effect on immune response markers.

The BARI-COVID is an open-label, non-randomized trial [55] to investigate the efficacy of baric prospective cohort, and 3 case control studies itinib in combination with antiviral treatments in hospitalized patients with mild to moderate COVID-19. It is expected to enroll 200 participants in Italy. The experimental arm participants will be given 4 mg baricitinib orally in combination with lopinavir/ritonavir once daily. Participants in the control arm will be given antiviral treatment or hydroxychloroquine for 2 weeks. Comparison of proportion of participants requiring ICU hospitalization and assessment of CRP, IL-6, and TNF levels are the primary endpoints.

BREATH [56], a pilot treatment trial in Italy, is an open label study to evaluate the safety and efficacy of oral baricitinib 4 mg for 7 days in hospitalized patients with COVID-19 pneumonia. There are no comparator or control arms. Measurement of oxygenation impairment (PaO_2/FiO_2) and mortality on day 8 are endpoints. On 15th day, assessment of the participants will be done for median SpO_2, number, types and severity of adverse events, biological assessments (level of various interleukins, TNF alpha, interferon gamma, viral load etc.) and rate of mortality.

Baricivid-19 [57], a phase II multicenter RCT in Italy, enrolled 126 patients (current status unclear) to compare baricitinib at a dose of 4 mg orally for 14 days (plus standard of care) against standard of care in hospitalized patients with COVID-19 pneumonia. The primary outcome is reduction in invasive ventilation at week 1 and 2, and there are multiple secondary endpoints like mortality (at 14, 28 days), time to invasive mechanical ventilation, length of hospital/ICU stays, toxicity.

Covid19COVINIB [58], an open label phase II RCT is proposed to enroll 165 patients to compare baricitinib and imatinib to supportive care therapy in patients with early COVID-19 pneumonia. The participants are designated to receive 400 mg OD of oral imatinib and 4 mg OD of oral baricitinib. Clinical improvement by at least two points on a 7-point ordinal scale is the primary end point, while safety (number of major side effects and early treatment cessation) and tolerability after 30 days are the secondary end points.

Another phase II trial is proposed in Canada, a non-randomized study on 800 adult patients hospitalized with moderate–severe COVID-19. Participants are to receive 2 mg oral baricitinib once day for 10 days, and the control arm would receive normal treatment. The primary objective of is to assess how long it takes for individuals to show clinical improvements in respiratory rate, fever, normal pulmonary function, and oxygen saturation.

The primary goal of the BARCOVID19 [60] trial in Spain is to ascertain the tolerability of baricitinib in oncohematological patients who have COVID-19 in phase I. It is anticipated that 136 participants will enroll in the trial. The aim of phase II of this trial is to establish if baricitinib (2–4 mg) reduces the inflammatory response caused by COVID-19, and prevents the development of severe ARDS in oncohematological patients as compared to other therapies given at the discretion of the investigator. Remdesivir or dexamethasone administration will be allowed if specific indications exist.

These ongoing clinical trials include different phases, randomized/non-randomized, single/multicentric studies in geographically diverse locations, with different doses of baricitinib. Indications include the different disease severities, and assessments are at varying timepoints or intervals for a plethora of COVID-19 related outcomes. However, the recruiting status of most of these trials is uncertain. Nevertheless, if evidence comes from these studies, it can be expected to be robust. The TACTIC-R platform trial in the UK is especially interesting, being a phase IV study, as baricitinib is still under review for approval of use in COVID-19 by the EMA [9], and its approval for COVID-19 in UK could not be found. The NICE recently approved the medication for moderate to severe atopic dermatitis in March 2021 [62]. Current knowledge about the Omicron variant of the SARS-CoV-2 virus is relatively limited in terms of its transmissibility, severity of disease as well as effectiveness of currently available vaccines and treatments including the newer treatments [63]. It has raised further question marks over the adequacy of treatment options available for management of COVID-19, for all grades of disease, and the apprehension towards new waves of the pandemic persists.

3.2 Current status of recommendation and limitations

In terms of the current status of recommendations for baricitinib in COVID-19 treatment, the US NIH COVID-19 treatment guidelines (February 2022) include baricitinib as an add-on treatment option to corticosteroids and/or remdesivir for hospitalized adult patients requiring oxygen or non-invasive ventilation, with the strength of recommendation being weak in patients requiring supplemental oxygen, and moderate in patients needing high flow oxygen or non-invasive ventilation [64]. It is also recommended that baricitinib not be used in combination with tocilizumab as both are potent immunosuppressants, leading to increased risk of infection. The WHO therapeutics and COVID-19 living guidelines have given strong recommendation (since January 2022) for the use of baricitinib as an alternative to IL-6 inhibitors in combination with corticosteroids in patients with severe or critical COVID-19, which includes hospitalized patients with $SpO_2 < 90\%$, signs of pneumonia, signs of severe respiratory distress, ARDS, sepsis /septic shock or requiring mechanical ventilation. However, baricitinib does not find a place as of now in the treatment recommendations/guidelines for COVID-19 from the UK-NICE or in countries like India, even though the drug has actually received an emergency approval in India [65, 66].

The qualitative synthesis of evidence that has been described in this chapter is quite comprehensive. But despite using the comprehensive WHO database of COVID research, a collection of most of the recognized electronic databases globally, for the literature search, there may still have been omissions especially from areas like gray or non-published literature. Majority of the studies finally selected were observational-mostly retrospective cohort, whereas only six published interventional studies could be found at the time of writing. In the hierarchy of evidence, observational studies are considered a relatively lower level of evidence. Non-uniformity of studies in terms of participants, outcomes, confounders etc. affects the external validity in the final analyses. As most of these studies are hospital based, a Berksonian bias is also likely to be present. The results of multiple clinical trials are not yet available as these are still ongoing or their current status is unknown.

4. Conclusion

Multiple observational and interventional studies published till date show that baricitinib used alone or in combination with other drugs, as an add-on to standard of care, reduces the mortality and producessignificant clinical improvements in patients hospitalized with severe to moderate COVID-19, particularly those requiring high flow oxygen or ventilation. Approval of the drug by the FDA for treatment of COVID-19 among hospitalized adults, as well as the strong recommendation by the WHO for its use as an add-on alternative option to be used in combination with corticosteroids, accurately justifies its current status as an established therapeutic approach for COVID-19.

Conflict of interest

None.

Notes/thanks/other declarations

None.

DOI: http://dx.doi.org/10.5772/intechopen.107269

Author details

Shubham Atal*, Ananyan Sampath, Aditya Banerjee and Ratinder Jhaj
All India Institute of Medical Sciences, Bhopal, Madhya Pradesh, India

*Address all correspondence to: shubham.pharm@aiimsbhopal.edu.in

References

[1] Coronavirus (COVID-19) Outbreak. World Health Organization. 2022. Available from: https://www.who.int/westernpacific/emergencies/covid-19. [Accessed: Dec 8, 2021]

[2] Huang C, Wang Y, Li X, Ren L, Zhao J, Hu Y, et al. Clinical features of patients infected with 2019 novel coronavirus in Wuhan, China. The Lancet (London, England). 2020;**395**:497-506. DOI: 10.1016/S0140-6736(20)30183-5

[3] Guidelines Development. COVID-19 Treat Guidelines n.d. National Institute of Health, Maryland, U.S.A. Available from: https://www.covid19treatmentguidelines.nih.gov/about-the-guidelines/guidelines-development/. [Accessed: Aug 4, 2022]

[4] Therapeutics and COVID-19: Living guideline. World Health Organization. 2022. Available from: https://www.who.int/publications/i/item/WHO-2019-nCoV-therapeutics-2022.4. [Accessed: Dec 9, 2021]

[5] EMA. COVID-19 treatments. The European Medicines Agency. 2021 https://www.ema.europa.eu/en/human-regulatory/overview/public-health-threats/coronavirus-disease-covid-19/treatments-vaccines/covid-19-treatments. [Accessed: Aug 2, 2022]

[6] Commissioner O of the. Coronavirus (COVID-19) Update: FDA Authorizes Drug Combination for Treatment of COVID-19. Maryland, U.S.A: U.S Food and Drug Administration; 2020. Available online: https://www.fda.gov/news-events/press-announcements/coronavirus-covid-19-update-fda-authorizes-drug-combination-treatment-covid-19. [Accessed June 8, 2021]

[7] Emergency Use Authorization (EUA) for baricitinib, FOR THE UNAPPROVED USE OF AN APPROVED PRODUCT Center for Drug Evaluation and Research (CDER) Review. U.S. Food and Drug Administration. 2022. Available from: https://www.fda.gov/media/158368/download. [Accessed: Sep 20, 2022]

[8] Baricitinib EUA. COVID-19 Emergency Use Authorization. Lilly. 2022. Available from: https://www.covid19.lilly.com/baricitinib/hcp. [Accessed: Sep 20, 2022]

[9] Pinho AC. EMA starts evaluating use of Olumiant in hospitalised COVID-19 patients requiring supplemental oxygen. European Medicines Agency. 2021. Available online: https://www.ema.europa.eu/en/news/ema-starts-evaluating-use-olumiant-hospitalised-covid-19-patients-requiring-supplemental-oxygen. [Accessed: Jun 8, 2021]

[10] Lilly accelerating baricitinib's availability in India following receipt of permission for restricted emergency use as a COVID-19 therapy via donations and licensing agreements. Eli Lilly and Company. 2022. Available from: https://investor.lilly.com/news-releases/news-release-details/lilly-accelerating-baricitinibs-availability-india-following. [Accessed: May 29, 2021]

[11] Markham A. Baricitinib: First global approval. Drugs. 2017;77:697-704. DOI: 10.1007/s40265-017-0723-3

[12] Gao Q, Liang X, Shaikh AS, Zang J, Xu W, Zhang Y. JAK/STAT signal transduction: Promising attractive targets for immune, inflammatory and hematopoietic diseases. Current Drug

Targets. 2018;**19**:487-500. DOI: 10.2174/1389450117666161207163054

[13] Damsky W, Peterson D, Ramseier J, Al-Bawardy B, Chun H, Proctor D, et al. The emerging role of Janus kinase inhibitors in the treatment of autoimmune and inflammatory diseases. The Journal of Allergy and Clinical Immunology. 2021;**147**:814-826. DOI: 10.1016/j.jaci.2020.10.022

[14] Mehta P, McAuley DF, Brown M, Sanchez E, Tattersall RS, Manson JJ. COVID-19: Consider cytokine storm syndromes and immunosuppression. The Lancet. 2020;**395**:1033-1034. DOI: 10.1016/S0140-6736(20)30628-0

[15] Cantini F, Niccoli L, Matarrese D, Nicastri E, Stobbione P, Goletti D. Baricitinib therapy in COVID-19: A pilot study on safety and clinical impact. The Journal of Infection. 2020;**81**:318-356. DOI: 10.1016/j.jinf.2020.04.017

[16] Cantini F, Niccoli L, Nannini C, Matarrese D, Natale MED, Lotti P, et al. Beneficial impact of Baricitinib in COVID-19 moderate pneumonia; multicentre study. The Journal of Infection. 2020;**81**:647-679. DOI: 10.1016/j.jinf.2020.06.052

[17] Seif F, Aazami H, Khoshmirsafa M, Kamali M, Mohsenzadegan M, Pornour M, et al. JAK inhibition as a new treatment strategy for patients with COVID-19. International Archives of Allergy and Immunology. 2020;**181**:467-475. DOI: 10.1159/000508247

[18] Spinelli FR, Conti F, Gadina M. HiJAKing SARS-CoV-2? The potential role of JAK inhibitors in the management of COVID-19. Science Immunology. 2020;**5**. DOI: 10.1126/sciimmunol.abc5367

[19] WHO COVID-19 Research Database. Global research on coronavirus disease (COVID-19). 2022. Available from: https://search.bvsalud.org/global-literature-on-novel-coronavirus-2019-ncov/. [Accessed: Jun 8, 2021]

[20] Clinical Spectrum of SARS-CoV-2 Infection. COVID-19 Treatment Guidelines. 2022. Available from: https://www.covid19treatmentguidelines.nih.gov/overview/clinical-spectrum/. [Accessed: Jun 8, 2021]

[21] Risk of bias tools - Current version of RoB 2. Creative Commons Attribution. 2022. Available from: https://www.riskofbias.info/welcome/rob-2-0-tool/current-version-of-rob-2. [Accessed: Jul 31, 2021]

[22] Study Quality Assessment Tools. National Heart, Lung and Blood Institute, National Institute of Health. 2022. Available from: https://www.nhlbi.nih.gov/health-topics/study-quality-assessment-tools. [Accessed: Jul 31, 2021]

[23] Hasan MJ, Rabbani R, Anam AM, Huq SMR, Polash MMI, Nessa SST, et al. Impact of high dose of baricitinib in severe COVID-19 pneumonia: A prospective cohort study in Bangladesh. BMC Infectious Diseases. 2021;**21**:427. DOI: 10.1186/s12879-021-06119-2

[24] Hasan MJ, Rabbani R, Anam AM, Huq SMR. Additional baricitinib loading dose improves clinical outcome in COVID-19. Open Medicine. 2021;**16**:041-046. DOI: 10.1515/med-2021-0010

[25] Titanji BK, Farley MM, Mehta A, Connor-Schuler R, Moanna A, Cribbs SK, et al. Use of Baricitinib in patients with moderate to severe coronavirus disease 2019. Clinical Infectious Diseases. 2021;**72**:1247-1250. DOI: 10.1093/cid/ciaa879

[26] Bronte V, Ugel S, Tinazzi E, Vella A, Sanctis FD, Canè S, et al. Baricitinib

restrains the immune dysregulation in patients with severe COVID-19. The Journal of Clinical Investigation. 2020;**130**:6409-6416. DOI: 10.1172/JCI141772

[27] Falcone M, Tiseo G, Barbieri G, Galfo V, Russo A, Virdis A, et al. Role of low-molecular-weight heparin in hospitalized patients with severe acute respiratory syndrome coronavirus 2 pneumonia: A prospective observational study. Open Forum Infectious Diseases. 2020;**7**(12):1-9. DOI: 10.1093/ofid/ofaa563

[28] Rosas J, Liaño FP, Cantó ML, Barea JMC, Beser AR, Rabasa JTA, et al. Experience with the use of Baricitinib and tocilizumab monotherapy or combined, in patients with interstitial pneumonia secondary to coronavirus COVID19: A real-world study. Reumatología Clínica. 2020;**18**(3):150-156. DOI: 10.1016/j.reuma.2020.10.009

[29] Milligan PS, Amsden J, Norris SA, Baker RL, Myers J, Preston F, et al. Clinical Outcomes in a Cohort of Non-Ventilated COVID-19 Patients with Progressive Hypoxemia and Hyper-Inflammatory Response Treated with Baricitinib. Rochester, NY: Social Science Research Network; 2020. DOI: 10.2139/ssrn.3594565

[30] Santos CS, Férnandez XC, Moriano Morales C, Álvarez ED, Álvarez Castro C, López Robles A, et al. Biological agents for rheumatic diseases in the outbreak of COVID-19: Friend or foe? RMD Open. 2021;7:e001439. DOI: 10.1136/rmdopen-2020-001439

[31] Pérez-Alba E, Nuzzolo-Shihadeh L, Aguirre-García GM, Espinosa-Mora J, Lecona-Garcia JD, Flores-Pérez RO, et al. Baricitinib plus dexamethasone compared to dexamethasone for the treatment of severe COVID-19 pneumonia: A retrospective analysis. Journal of Microbiology, Immunology, and Infection = Wei mian yu gan ran za zhi. 2021;**54**:787-793. DOI: 10.1016/j.jmii.2021.05.009

[32] Amarnath A, Das A, Mutya V, Ibrahim I. The Effect of Baricitinib Usage on the Clinical and Biochemical Profiles of Covid-19 Patients—A Retrospective Observational Study. Cold Spring Harbor Laboratory; 2021. DOI: 10.1101/2021.08.11.21261760

[33] García-García JA, Pérez-Quintana M, Ramos-Giráldez C, Cebrián-González I, Martín-Ponce ML, Del Valle-Villagrán J, et al. Anakinra versus Baricitinib: Different strategies for patients hospitalized with COVID-19. Journal of Clinical Medicine. 2021;**10**:4019. DOI: 10.3390/jcm10174019

[34] Rodriguez-Garcia JL, Sanchez-Nievas G, Arevalo-Serrano J, Garcia-Gomez C, Jimenez-Vizuete JM, Martinez-Alfaro E. Baricitinib improves respiratory function in patients treated with corticosteroids for SARS-CoV-2 pneumonia: An observational cohort study. Rheumatology. 2021;**60**:399-407. DOI: 10.1093/rheumatology/keaa587

[35] Iglesias Gómez R, Méndez R, Palanques-Pastor T, Ballesta-López O, Borrás Almenar C, Megías Vericat JE, et al. Baricitinib against severe COVID-19: Effectiveness and safety in hospitalised pretreated patients. European Journal of Hospital Pharmacy: Science and Practice. 2021;**29**(e1):e41-e45. DOI: 10.1136/ejhpharm-2021-002741

[36] Abizanda P, Calbo Mayo JM, Mas Romero M, Cortés Zamora EB, Tabernero Sahuquillo MT, Romero Rizos L, et al. Baricitinib reduces 30-day mortality in older adults with moderate-to-severe COVID-19 pneumonia. Journal of the American Geriatrics Society. 2021;**69**:2752-2758. DOI: 10.1111/jgs.17357

[37] Thoms BL, Gosselin J, Libman B, Littenberg B, Budd R. Efficacy of combination therapy with the JAK inhibitor Baricitinib In the treatment of COVID-19. Research Square. 2021. DOI: 10.21203/rs.3.rs-835734/v1

[38] Perez-Gutierrez V, Shah V, Afzal A, Khalid A, Yangco A, Ocrospoma S, et al. Combination of Baricitinib plus Remdesivir and Dexamethasone improves time to recovery and mortality among hospitalized patients with severe COVID-19 infection. Cold Spring Harbor Laboratory. medRxiv. 2022. DOI: 10.1101/2022.04.04.22273425

[39] Tanimoto T, Tada S, Fujita S, Hirakawa T, Matsumura M, Isoyama S, et al. Effect of baricitinib in patients with coronavirus disease 2019 and respiratory failure: A propensity score-matched retrospective cohort study. Respiratory Investigation. 2022;**60**:418-424. DOI: 10.1016/j.resinv.2022.02.004

[40] Yasuda Y, Hirayama Y, Uemasu K, Arasawa S, Iwashima D, Takahashi K. Efficacy of the combination of baricitinib, remdesivir, and dexamethasone in hypoxic adults with COVID-19: A retrospective study. Respiratory Medicine and Research. 2022;**81**:100903. DOI: 10.1016/j.resmer.2022.100903

[41] So JM, Umeh C, Noriega S, Stratton E, Aseri M, Gupta RC. Use of Baricitinib in combination with remdesivir and steroid in COVID-19 treatment: A multicenter retrospective study. Cureus. 2021;**13**. DOI: 10.7759/cureus.20620

[42] Bryushkova E, Skatova V, Mutovina Z, Zagrebneva A, Fomina D, Kruglova T, et al. Tocilizumab, netakimab, and baricitinib in patients with mild-to-moderate COVID-19: An observational study. PLOS ONE. 2022;**13**(12):e20620

[43] Tziolos N, Karofylakis E, Grigoropoulos I, Kazakou P, Koullias E, Savva A, et al. Real-life effectiveness and safety of Baricitinib as adjunctive to standard-of-care treatment in hospitalized patients with severe coronavirus disease 2019. Open Forum Infectious Diseases. 2022;**9**:ofab588. DOI: 10.1093/ofid/ofab588

[44] Hasan MJ, Rabbani R, Anam AM, Huq SMR. Therapeutic safety and efficacy of triple-immunosuppressants versus dual-immunosuppressants in severe-to-critical COVID-19: A prospective cohort study in Bangladesh. Annals of Medicine. 2022;**54**:723-732. DOI: 10.1080/07853890.2022.2039958

[45] Marconi V, Ramanan A, de Bono S, Kartman C, Krishnan V, Liao R et al. Efficacy and safety of baricitinib for the treatment of hospitalised adults with COVID-19 (COV-BARRIER): A randomised, double-blind, parallel-group, placebo-controlled phase 3 trial. The Lancet Respiratory Medicine. 2021;**9**:1407-1418. DOI: 10.1101/2021.04.30.21255934

[46] Frost MT, Jimenez-Solem E, Ankarfeldt MZ, Nyeland ME, Andreasen AH, Petersen TS. The adaptive COVID-19 treatment trial-1 (ACTT-1) in a real-world population: A comparative observational study. Critical Care (London, England). 2020;**24**:677. DOI: 10.1186/s13054-020-03406-3

[47] Kalil AC, Patterson TF, Mehta AK, Tomashek KM, Wolfe CR, Ghazaryan V, et al. Baricitinib plus remdesivir for hospitalized adults with Covid-19. The New England Journal of Medicine. 2021;**384**:795-807. DOI: 10.1056/NEJMoa2031994

[48] Izumo T, Kuse N, Awano N, Tone M, Sakamoto K, Takada K, et al. Clinical

impact of combination therapy with baricitinib, remdesivir, and dexamethasone in patients with severe COVID-19. Respiratory Investigation. 2021;**59**:799-803. DOI: 10.1016/j.resinv.2021.07.004

[49] Gavriilidis E, Antoniadou C, Chrysanthopoulou A, Ntinopoulou M, Smyrlis A, Fotiadou I, et al. Combined administration of inhaled DNase, baricitinib and tocilizumab as rescue treatment in COVID-19 patients with severe respiratory failure. Clinical Immunology. 2022;**238**:109016

[50] Ely EW, Ramanan AV, Kartman CE, de Bono S, Liao R, MLB P, et al. Baricitinib plus standard of care for hospitalised adults with COVID-19 on invasive mechanical ventilation or extracorporeal membrane oxygenation: Results of a randomised. Placebo-Controlled Trial. 2021. DOI: 10.1101/2021.10.11.21263897

[51] Wolfe CR, Tomashek KM, Patterson TF, Gomez CA, Marconi VC, Jain MK, et al. Baricitinib versus dexamethasone for adults hospitalised with COVID-19 (ACTT-4): A randomised, double-blind, double placebo-controlled trial. The Lancet Respiratory Medicine. 2022;**10**(9):888-899. DOI: 10.1016/S2213-2600(22)00088-1

[52] Kulkarni S, Fisk M, Kostapanos M, Banham-Hall E, Bond S, Hernan-Sancho E, et al. Repurposed immunomodulatory drugs for Covid-19 in pre-ICu patients - mulTi-Arm Therapeutic study in pre-ICu patients admitted with Covid-19 – Repurposed Drugs (TACTIC-R): A structured summary of a study protocol for a randomised controlled trial. Trials. 2020;**21**:626

[53] Tombetti E. Factorial, multicentric, randomized clinical trial of remdesivir and immunotherapy in combination with dexamethasone for moderate COVID-19 (the AMMURAVID trial). Clinicaltrials.gov. 2021

[54] Cumulative adaptive, multiarm, multistage and multicentre randomized clinical trial with immunotherapy for Moderate COVID-19. Clinicaltrialsregister.eu. 2022. Available from: https://www.clinicaltrialsregister.eu/ctr-search/trial/2020-001854-23/IT. [Accessed: Jul 3, 2021]

[55] Cantini F. Baricitinib combined with antiviral therapy in symptomatic patients infected by COVID-19: An open-label, Pilot Study. Clinicaltrials.gov. 2020

[56] Baricitinib for coRona Virus pnEumonia (COVID-19): A THerapeutic Trial—Full Text View. ClinicalTrials.gov. Clinicaltrials.gov. 2022. Available from: https://clinicaltrials.gov/ct2/show/NCT04399798. [Accessed: Jul 21, 2021]

[57] Menichetti F. BARICIVID-19 Study: MultiCentre, randomised, phase IIa clinical trial evaluating efficacy and tolerability of Baricitinib as add-on treatment of in-patients with COVID-19 compared to standard therapy. Clinicaltrials.gov. 2020

[58] Hospital Universitario de Fuenlabrada. Prospective, phase II, randomized, open-label, parallel group study to evaluate the efficacy of Baricitinib, imatinib or supportive treatment in patients with SARS Cov2 pneumonia. Clinicaltrials.gov. 2021

[59] Barrett L. Treatment of moderate to severe coronavirus disease (COVID-19) in hospitalized patients. Clinicaltrials.gov. 2020

[60] Moreno-González G, Mussetti A, Albasanz-Puig A, Salvador I, Sureda A,

Gudiol C, et al. A phase I/II clinical trial to evaluate the efficacy of baricitinib to prevent respiratory insufficiency progression in onco-hematological patients affected with COVID19: A structured summary of a study protocol for a randomised controlled trial. Trials. 2021;**22**:116. DOI: 10.1186/s13063-021-05072-4

[61] Kulkarni S, Fisk M, Kostapanos M, Banham-Hall E, Bond S, Hernan-Sancho E, et al. Repurposed immunomodulatory drugs for Covid-19 in pre-ICu patients—mulTi-arm therapeutic study in pre-ICu patients admitted with Covid-19—Repurposed drugs (TACTIC-R): A structured summary of a study protocol for a randomised controlled trial. Trials. 2020;**21**:626. DOI: 10.1186/s13063-020-04535-4

[62] Baricitinib for treating moderate to severe atopic dermatitis- Guidance. National Institute for Health and Care Excellence. 2022. Available from: https://www.nice.org.uk/guidance/ta681. [Accessed: December 9, 2021]

[63] Update on Omicron. WHO. Available from: https://www.who.int/news/item/28-11-2021-update-on-omicron. [Accessed: Dec 9, 2021]

[64] Therapeutic Management of Hospitalized Adults With COVID-19. COVID-19 Treatment Guidelines. National Institute of Health. 2022. Available from: https://www.covid19treatmentguidelines.nih.gov/management/clinical-management-of-adults/hospitalized-adults--therapeutic-management/. [Accessed: Dec 9, 2021]

[65] Therapeutics and COVID-19: Living Guideline. WHO. 2022. Available from: https://www.who.int/publications-detail-redirect/WHO-2019-nCoV-therapeutics-2022.4. [Accessed: August 2, 2022]

[66] Revised guidelines for Home Isolation of mild/asymptomatic COVID-19 cases. Ministry of Health & Family Welfare, Government of India. 2022. Available from: https://www.mohfw.gov.in/pdf/Revised Illustrated GuidelinesforHomeIsolationof MildAsymptomaticCOVID19 Cases.pdf. [Accessed: Aug 4, 2022]

Chapter 4

New Perspective and Applications of Homeopathy in Treating COVID-19 Symptoms

Ameya Sharma, Sandeep Puri, Varun Puri, Divya Dheer, Neha Bhandari and Vivek Puri

Abstract

The long-term effects of infections such as COVID-19 survivor therapy and post-coronavirus infection are still being researched. The severe acute respiratory syndrome (SARS-CoV-2)-caused new coronavirus disease (COVID-19) outbreak is seeing a significant increase in affected individuals worldwide. In severe and critical COVID-19 patients, SARS-CoV-2 has been demonstrated to disrupt normal immunological responses, resulting in a weakened immune system and uncontrolled inflammatory reactions. Lymphocytic activation and dysfunction, granulocyte and monocyte abnormalities, elevated cytokine levels, and a rise in immunoglobulin G (IgG) and total antibodies are all seen in these patients. Scientists from all over the world are working constantly to identify particular treatments and vaccinations for Covid-19. Several cases of treatment have been recorded by homeopathic practitioners around the world, with encouraging results. Bryonia alba, Phosphorus, Arsenic album, Gelsemium sempervirens, and Camphora are some of the Homeopathic medicines that have shown to be effective. Government of India (Ministry of AYUSH) has promoted and approved Arsenic album 30 as an immune booster for its potential involvement in preventing COVID-19, and findings are gradually favoring for this drug. In the management of post-COVID-19 outcomes, homeopathy drugs can be used to treat non-COVID conditions. We explored new perspectives and applications of homeopathic medications that can help with COVID and post-COVID symptoms in this chapter.

Keywords: homeopathy, COVID-19, AYUSH, case study, applications

1. Introduction

After first appearing in Wuhan, China, in late December 2019, the severe acute respiratory syndrome coronavirus 2 (SARS CoV-2) quickly spread throughout the world [1, 2]. The severity of COVID-19 symptoms can range from a self-limiting respiratory disease to severe progressive pneumonia, multiorgan failure, and death [3–7]. Despite extensive research and numerous ongoing clinical trials [8], there are currently no effective therapeutic medicines for treating or curing a coronavirus infection. Pathological characteristics of SARS-CoV-2 of the family Coronaviridae, which have an RNA genome with a 5′ methylation cap and a 3′ polyadenylated tail, allowing the RNA to connect to ribosomes for translation [9, 10]. The replicase protein encoded by coronavirus genomes facilitates RNA viral genome transcription into new RNA copies by leveraging the host cell's machinery. The protease-like non-structural protein found in coronaviruses can rupture the protein chain [11, 12]. A surge in type 2 cytokines and a decline in T-cell and B-cell activity that intensifies with age [13] may indicate a poor prognosis for patients with COVID-19.

According to the World Health Organization (WHO), the combination drug Paxlovid (nirmatrelvir and ritonavir) is the best therapeutic choice for high-risk patients with mild to moderate COVID-19 who are at highest risk of hospital admission. Patients with mild COVID-19 who are at the most risk of developing severe disease and hospitalization, such as the unvaccinated, the elderly, and the immunosuppressed, are highly encouraged to use Pfizer's oral antiviral medication (a combination of nirmatrelvir and ritonavir tablets). New evidence from two randomized controlled trials involving 3078 participants supports this recommendation. According to the numbers, this treatment decreases the likelihood of hospitalization by 85%. This translates to 84% fewer hospitalizations per 1000 patients in the high-risk group (those with a probability of hospitalization of 10% or above) [14].

The use of homeopathy is widespread in every WHO Region. Use of homeopathic medications, largely as over-the-counter medicines, is increasing in many regions of the world, despite differences in the national regulatory structure and the status of homeopathy within the health care system. While there is some uncertainty about the extent of the homeopathic medicines industry, sales figures indicate that homeopathic medications constitute a large part of medical markets.

Homeopathic remedies, or the stocks or mother tinctures from which they are made, are derived from either naturally occurring or manufactured ingredients that are listed in pharmacopoeial monographs or other legally recognized sources. The following are examples of possible ingredients in homeopathic remedies (excluding imponderables): Animal materials include whole animals, animal organs, tissues, secretions, cell lines, poisons, nosodes, blood products; Plant materials including roots, stems, leaves, flowers, bark, pollen, lichen, moss, ferns, and algae; Microorganisms including fungi, bacteria, viruses, and plant parasites; Tissues, secretions, cell lines, and endogenous chemicals like hormones are all examples of human materials; elements of nature and synthetic chemicals.

It is important that the source materials and excipients used to make homeopathic medicines are of good quality. Some homeopathic remedies contain ingredients whose usage is prohibited in conventional medicine due to safety concerns. To put it simply, nosodes are diluted versions of pathogenic organs or tissues; infectious agents like bacteria, fungus, eggs, parasites, virus particles, and yeast; illness products like excretions or secretions; or anything else that can cause an infection. There is always a chance that anything made with human or animal parts is contaminated with disease-causing organisms. Some homeopathic remedies have poisonous animal or plant ingredients, while others, especially when taken in their fresh form, can quickly degrade or get contaminated by microorganisms.

Heavy metals and insecticides may be present in plant materials. Plants can have widely varying levels of hazardous compounds. Guidelines for Good Manufacturing Practice (GMP) regarding the manufacturing process, facilities, staff, packaging, and labeling are applicable to both conventional and homeopathic drugs. Misidentification, impurity of starting material, cross-contamination, and inadvertent contamination are just a few of the quality and safety issues that can arise from a lack of GMP. There are a number of specific consequences that require specially qualified and experienced workers due to the unique characteristics of homeopathic medicine production. These are the facilities that deal with homeopathic medications originating from animal or human origins, as well as poisonous materials and materials (especially fresh ones) that are susceptible to degradation processes and microbial contamination. Accidental or intentional contamination of source materials, excipients, or diluents, or the vessel or bottle used to make the dilution, might affect the characteristics of homeopathic medications. The final homeopathic medicines might vary significantly due to differences in definitions among pharmacopeias as well as in the processing procedures and manufacturing methods used to manufacture them [15].

As with conventional pharmaceuticals, homeopathic remedies must comply with the provisions of the Federal Food, Drug, and Cosmetic Act pertaining to approval, adulteration, and misbranding. As of right now, the FDA has not authorized the sale of any homeopathic remedies.

The FDA's enforcement policy on homeopathic medicines was laid down in Compliance Policy Guide (CPG) 400.400, "Conditions Under Which Homeopathic Drugs May Be Marketed," published in 1988. Due to inconsistency with our risk-based strategy to regulatory and enforcement action, FDA removed CPG 400.400 on October 24, 2019. Drug Products Labeled as Homeopathic: Revised Draft Guidance was also released by FDA for public feedback. The FDA has not given its stamp of approval to any homeopathic drug on the market, so it's possible that these items do not measure up to today's rigorous quality, safety, and efficacy criteria. To address the issue of unapproved homeopathic remedies in the market, this updated proposed advice suggests a risk-based enforcement strategy [16].

A survey of 293 general practitioners in the Netherlands found that 45% of them think that homeopathic remedies are effective for treating upper respiratory tract infections or hay fever. However, many medical practitioners reject homeopathy as a viable therapeutic option due to the highly improbable notion that drugs diluted to such an extreme degree still retain their biological effects. Furthermore, it is frequently asserted that modern procedures, such as controlled studies, have not been used to assess the efficacy of homeopathy. Synthesis based on predetermined criteria showed methodological quality analysis of 107 randomized controlled trials published in 96 papers. The quality of the trials was evaluated using a predetermined set of criteria, and the results were interpreted in context of the trials' quality. There were 14 trials examining the efficacy of classical homeopathy, and another 58 trials in which patients with similar conventional diagnoses were all given the same homeopathic treatment. In 26 trials, various homeopathic treatment combinations were examined, while in 9 trials, isopathic treatment was examined. There were many high-quality trials among what appeared to be mostly poor ones. There was a generally good pattern of findings, and this held true regardless of the quality of the trials or the type of homeopathy that was employed. A total of 81 studies showing favorable results and 24 trials showing no positive effects of homeopathy were found out of 105 trials having interpretable results [17].

For almost two centuries, people with all sorts of ailments have turned to homeopathy for relief. Homeopathy has a long history of successfully treating epidemic diseases through prevention and treatment, and its efficacy has been demonstrated in clinical trials, meta-analyses, and systematic reviews [18–20]. While some people may see homeopathy favorably, it remains a highly contentious kind of complementary and alternative medicine. Two different theories form its basis. First, the idea that a drug that creates the same symptoms in healthy people can also cure the disease it is meant to treat. Furthermore, "the law of minimum dose" states that the smaller the dosage, the greater the therapeutic impact [21, 22]. When it comes to homeopathy, it's not like one drug cures one illness. Instead, it is a method in which treatments are tailored to specific patients based on overarching patterns and unique qualities revealed by an exhaustive analysis of all of the patient's reported physical, mental, and emotional distress. Public health measures like as social isolation, hand washing, face covering, and quarantine are now the only preventative treatments available in conventional medicine [23]. The use of homeopathic methods for disease prevention is widespread across the globe. When it comes to homeopathic medicine, *Arsenicum album* is highly recommended by the Indian Ministry of AYUSH (Ayurveda, Yoga and Naturopathy, Unani, Siddha, and Homeopathy) [24]. With regards to treatment, the homeopathic community suggested gathering cases to evaluate and validate appropriate homeopathic treatment for the COVID-19 pandemic before more extensive, systematic investigations were done [25, 26]. Homeopathy [27] is being studied as a potential treatment for SARS-CoV-2 [28] in clinical trials. Several encouraging studies have shown that homeopathic medicines for COVID-19 symptoms have a high success rate. In this chapter, we will primarily focus on the evidence from clinical studies, novel perspectives, and applications of homeopathic treatments for COVID-19 symptoms [29].

2. Clinical presentation and diagnostic procedure

As of now, we know that most people infected with COVID-19 will experience only mild to moderate symptoms after an incubation period of 1–14 days, and that most of these people will recover without any additional therapy at all. However, numerous asymptomatic infected people have been identified, and each of them could develop symptoms and spread the disease [30, 31]. Infection with the COVID-19 virus typically causes fever, dry cough, and throat pain/itching. Body aches, headaches, and shortness of breath are among possible symptoms, along with diarrhea, nausea, and a runny nose. Laboratory testing for COVID-19 is necessary for making a definitive diagnosis. This can be done by verifying the presence of the virus or by examining the specific antibodies developed in response to infection. Initial screening for the coronavirus is recommended by the majority of countries by using reverse transcription polymerase chain reaction (RT-PCR). A positive result from this test indicates that an infection is either extremely recent or is still ongoing. Nasopharyngeal swabs and sputum samples are examples of respiratory samples that can be tested. In addition, the identification of particular antibodies (serology) is helpful for diagnosis and population surveillance, especially in the later stages of the infection [30, 32].

3. Homeopathic approach towards COVID-19 symptoms

Currently, hospital-based risk management and symptomatic treatment are the only options for COVID-19. Due to its symptom-focused approach, the homeopathic medical system can be an effective tool in the fight against this worldwide epidemic. In the event of an epidemic or pandemic, the first line of defense is to take precautions by teaching the public how to protect themselves from infection and by providing interventions that will maintain their natural immunity. According to the Advisory from the Ministry of AYUSH, homeopaths are encouraged to inform the public about Genus epidemicus that has been identified by designated specialists as beneficial for improving immunity. Numerous homeopathic medications, including *Arsenic Album, Pulsatilla, Silicia, Natrum Muriaticum, Phosphorus, Calcarea Carbonicum, Hepar Sulfur, Lachesis, Nux Vomica, Sulfur*, and many others, are available for patients with COVID-19 infection [33, 34].

The second approach is to provide affected people with homeopathic symptomatic mitigation [35]. It has been shown that homeopathic medicines can be effective in treating infectious disorders such as the Influenza-like illness, dengue, and acute encephalitis syndrome. The ability of homeopathic medications to modulate the immune system has also been demonstrated in several published preclinical investigations. Depending on the severity of the individual situation, these medications may be provided together or separately [36, 37].

4. Efficiency of homeopathy in epidemic

Even before the widespread use of modern sanitation, vaccination, and antibiotics, the homeopathic medical system has developed protocols for the management of infectious outbreaks. Hahnemann utilized *Belladonna* to stop an epidemic of scarlet fever in Europe in the year 1799 AD, and he reported his findings in a treatise [33, 38]. *Aconite*, another homeopathic medication, was shown to be effective against the Scarlet fever epidemic that ravaged Germany between the years 1800 AD and 1808 AD. *Bryonia alba, Hyoscyamus niger, or Rhus Toxicodendron* (singly or regularly) were all effective treatments for the typhoid outbreak that hit Europe in 1813 AD [39]. In 1831 AD., he wrote about the use of *camphor, cuprum metallicum, and veratrum album* as Genus Epidemicus for preventing and treating pandemics from Asia in the Germanic territory. *Camphor* was one of his recommended preventative medicines for the infection, while *Cuprum metallicum or Veratrum album* were recommended for later stages of infection [40]. Success in treating epidemics with homeopathic medications including typhoid, cholera, yellow fever, scarlet fever, smallpox, diphtheria, Spanish flu, meningitis, and polio made homeopathy popular in the United States and Europe in the nineteenth century [38, 41]. Full case analysis is performed before a patient is prescribed medicine in homeopathy. Patients impacted by an epidemic typically have similar symptoms. If the same drug is prescribed to multiple patients after the analysis, the drug may be labeled as the "Genus Epidemicus" drug for that geographical area. Within a few days of a pandemic outbreak, this should be decided. Hahnemann discovered interesting differences between epidemic strains of illness. Hahnemann highlighted in his article "Observations on the Scarlet Fever" [42] that there is no assurance that medications taken in earlier epidemics will be effective in the next outbreak. In the sixth edition of his book, "the Organon of Medicine," Dr. Hahnemann made specific reference to the choice of "homoeopathic (specific) medicine" in Aphorisms 102 (footnotes), 147, and 241. Using this strategy, Cuba eradicated Kerato conjunctivitis in 1995, and India eradicated Chikungunya in Kerala in 2007 [38]. Other Cuban researchers showed that homeoprophylaxis was helpful in preventing leptospirosis when it was provoked by extensive hurricane damage in 2007 and 2008 [43]. There are several typical cold-like symptoms described by those infected with COVID-19. As a result, homeopathic doctors have decided to treat patients with COVID-19 with the same medication and dosage that is recommended for patients suffering from the common cold. Some few over-the-counter medications that have been effective in treating individuals with the common cold and COVID-19 are discussed below.

4.1 Aspidosperma

Alleviate asthma symptoms for many individuals; by doing so, it raises blood oxygen levels and stimulates the respiratory centers; the symptom of "wanting to breathe" during exercising is the primary indicator; the condition is called cardiac asthma; pulmonary stenosis, infarction of the pulmonary artery due to thrombosis [29].

4.2 Arsenic album

An extremely effective treatment for all of the body's organs and tissues; deadliness and septic diseases; distress and unrest on a grand scale; extremely thirsty; consumes large volumes of liquid in frequent, little doses; acid reflux is characterized by the reflexive ingestion of acidic or bitter substances that appear to irritate the lining of the throat; swollen and painful liver and spleen; shooting discomfort in the right upper lobe of the lung; cannot sleep because you are afraid of suffocating; limitations on breathing space midnight is when asthma attacks peak; aching in the middle of my chest; intense heat; adynamia is a sign of periodicity; infected fevers intermittent; incomplete paroxysms accompanied by extreme fatigue [25, 44, 45].

4.3 Pulsatilla

Even though it's cold outside, the patient prefers to be in the fresh air; dry mouthed, grumpy, and shivering; exudates that are viscous, tasteless, and pale greenish; chronically shifting symptoms; prone to frequent tears; enjoys being shown compassion; having coryza means that your right nostril is blocked and you are experiencing pain at the base of your nose; smell impairment; lack of saliva and thirst; desire for regular mouth washings; a habitual licker of dry lips; dislikes warm or fatty foods and beverages; morning loose cough followed by dry nighttime cough that requires sitting up in bed to alleviate; venous distention and unbearable heat make going outside a miserable experience; a headache, diarrhea, loss of appetite, and nausea are all symptoms that occur during apyrexia [25, 46].

4.4 Silicea

Suppurative processes; adverse reactions to vaccinations. mindful and physical submission; a high susceptibility to getting sick from the cold; children that are stubborn and willful; dizziness from staring upwards; best to bundle up itchy, watery eyes in the morning; having trouble smelling and eventually losing that ability; hair-on-the-tongue feeling; stabbing like a pin in the tonsil; feeling of a cold settling into the throat; eruption of the parotid glands; a sharp discomfort when swallowing; coughing fits when lying down; expectoration is thick and yellow and lumpy; feelings of chill in the limbs even when indoors; nighttime sweating that gets worse in the morning; areas of the body that are suffering are ice cold [47].

4.5 Natrum muriaticum

Sensation of tightness all over the body; dryness of the mucous membranes; negative reactions to negative emotions such as grief, fear, wrath, etc.; extreme fatigue and weakness excruciating pain; tears roll down your face when you cough, and waking up in the morning feels like a thousand tiny hammers are hammering on your forehead. Watery, thin discharge, like the white of a raw egg; never fails to prevent the onset of a cold; the inability to smell or taste; mapping the tongue; relax from 9 am until 11 am; temperature; fever causes an increase in thirst; fever-blisters; feelings of chilliness all over the body that do not seem to go away [48, 49].

4.6 Phosphorus

In addition to irritating and inflaming mucous membranes and serous membranes, *phosphorus* can also induce their degeneration. Rapid onset of symptoms, including fainting, sweating, and falling to the ground suicide anxiety when alone; skin that looks painfully pale, with blue circles beneath the eyes; the hippocratic oath; need ice cold water badly; esophageal narrowing; produces copious amounts of vomit after eating; getting sick; throwing up water once it warms up in the stomach. Tickling in the throat causes coughing; exposure to cold air, reading, laughing, or talking makes it worse. Feeling of heaviness or pressure in the chest. Painful, stabbing sensation in the chest; rapid, stifled breathing it feel like there is a fire going in the chest; suffocating pneumonitis; laying on one's left side is far worse; body-wide trembling and coughing; in the evenings, the Sputa is rusty and cold. Aching knees after a long day; unmoving due to lack of thirst but with an abnormal appetite [50, 51].

4.7 Calcarea carbonicum

It treats the twitching cough, the brief chest pains, the nausea, the stomach acid, and the aversion to fat; lacks stamina and fatigues quickly; relapses are common, and recovery time is disrupted; extreme sensitivity to the cold; occasional sweating children have a penchant for eggs, but they also consume dirt and other indigestible substances. Patients with *calcarea* are typically large, pale, flabby, and sweaty, as well as chilly, moist, and sour. Hoarseness that is not painful, but is worse in the morning, and a tickling cough that's most bothersome at night. Only daytime expectoration is permitted; viscous mucus that is yellow in color and has a sour taste; extreme sensitivity to percussion and touch in the chest; seeking to get some air; at 2:00 p.m., a chill spreads across the stomach region; flu-like symptoms, including sweating; strong and regular heartbeats [52, 53].

4.8 Hepar sulfur

Those with a scrofulous or lymphatic constitution, who are more prone to breakouts and swelling of the glands, will benefit the most from this; experiencing a gust of wind in an area; even a minor provocation can set him off; corner-of-the-mouth ulcers; you feel like there's a splinter or a blockage in your throat whenever you try to swallow; quinsy, with suppuration in the horizon; suffering from swallowing-inducing stitches that go all the way to the ear; trapping mucus; coughing fits brought on by exposure to cold, especially while eating anything cold; loose, rattling cough from croup; symptoms are greater in the morning; coughing so hard that you cannot breathe; cold when exposed to air or even a gentle breeze; excessive nighttime dry heat; heavy perspiration; a putrid, disagreeable stench [50, 54].

4.9 Lachesis

Feeling of strain in various areas; cannot take a tight grip on anything; prodigious fluency in speech; patches of aphthous dermatitis and bareness, with pain and redness; bad flavor; worse on the left side, and it hurts to drink liquids; experiencing quinsy; discomfort made worse by hot beverages; extremely distressing; the smallest pressure, the slightest contact, is excruciating. It's important that the collar and neck-band be quite slack; frequent dry, suffocating, and irritating coughing; having low secretion and a high degree of sensitivity; laryngeal irritation made worse by open air and the lack of a pillow; shivering shoulders, freezing toes, a blazing flush, and a burning sweat; acids cause a recurrence of paroxysm; recurring springtime fever with intermittent symptoms [53, 55].

4.10 Nux vomica

Nux patients tend to be slender, frail, fast, lively, tense, and irritable; irritated by any external stimulus; avoids physical contact; having a headache outside in the bright sun; symptoms of a cold or the flu made worse by being indoors in a warm environment. Exudation that is acrid but accompanied by a sense of congestion; a sensation of being scratched and rubbed raw; having a good morning tickle; a feeling of tightness, stress, or roughness; bloated feeling in the upper abdomen (epigastrium) and the pressure of a stone some hours after eating; full stomach and asthma, especially in the morning or after eating; coughing, with the feeling that something has been pulled loose in the chest; poor lung capacity; limited capacity for respiration; a high degree of strictness, as evidenced by blue fingernails; abdominal pain and generalized aches and pains; fever stages are cold; always wear layers. Feelings of chilliness when exposed, despite his refusal to wear clothing; internal dry heat [25, 56].

4.11 Sulfur

Extreme heat, aversion to water, dry skin and hair, reddened genitalia, nausea and vomiting around 11 a.m., and catnaps; for *sulfur* patients, standing is the worst possible position; *sulfur* subjects almost invariably exhibit irritability, depression, emaciation, and weakness while having a healthy appetite. Itchy, red, and scaly skin that bleeds easily; chronic dry catarrh adenoids and polyps; feelings of tightness and heat in the chest; respiratory distress; prefers an open window middle-of-the-night dyspnea that is alleviated by sitting up; morning heart rate is higher than nighttime heart rate; greenish, purulent, pleasant expectoration; coughing worse when conversing or in the morning; bursts of intense heat; rapid and severe rises in core body temperature; excruciating parchingness and thirst; night perspiration (especially around the nape and occiput); localized perspiration (especially on the hands and feet); smelly perspiration; spontaneous, intermittent, and relapsing [50, 52].

4.12 Bryonia

Dryness of the mucous membranes; when the *bryonia* patient raises their head, they have dizziness and a pressive headache, and they are agitated. Chapped, cracked lips and tongue; an abnormally high need to urinate, a distaste for most foods, a hypersensitive epigastric region, and an uncomfortable sensation of having a stone lodged in one's stool that is dry and firm; a dry cough; *Bryonia* has a propensity for leanness and irritability, and it has the most noticeable effects on people whose constitutions already include sturdy, firm fiber and dark skin. It acts most visibly on the right side, in the evening, and in the open air, especially after a cold spell; hacking cough that makes you feel like your chest is going to explode; rapid, laboured breathing made worse by physical exertion; this condition is the result of chest sutures. Shiver with a dry cough and sutures; radiant warmth from within; sour perspiration after even mild exercise; an abundance of sweating that is simple to induce; gastric and liver problems are markers of rheumatic and typhoid fever [52, 57].

4.13 Vanadium metallicum

Utilized in cases of anemia and other forms of wasting illness due to its oxygen-carrying and catalytic properties; in addition to increasing hemoglobin levels, this process combines oxygen from the blood with the toxines, neutralizing them; anxiety that spreads throughout the chest; dry, irritating, and paroxysmal cough, which may be accompanied by bleeding; nasal, ocular, and pharyngeal irritation [58].

5. Case study

Randomized clinical studies, which are designed to examine how one medication cures one condition with one primary outcome, are unsuitable for investigating homeopathic remedies because of their subjectivity and individuality [59]. All COVID-19 patients with RT-PCR confirmation, received home isolation and care at COVID Care Centers. Patients with minimal to moderate illness were all taken into account. In the mildest cases, patients had simple upper respiratory tract infections and showed no signs of respiratory discomfort or oxygen deprivation (normal oxygen saturation). Patients with a respiratory rate more than or equal to 24 breaths per minute and an oxygen saturation (SpO2) of less than 94% (range: 90–94%) on room air were identified as having moderate pneumonia [28, 60]. Patients with multiple medical conditions were also included.

Patients were checked on once a day for up to a week or until their symptoms subsided completely. Patients who were quarantined at home were called daily to monitor on their condition. As with any frequent follow-up of a homeopathic case, the patient was questioned about the severity of their symptoms and their general health at each visit. At each follow-up, patients were rated on a scale from −4 to +4 called the Outcome in Relation to Impact on Daily Living (ORIDL) [61].

Establishing causality between medication and improved health is a major obstacle in prognostic factor research, as the cure could be the result of the homeopathic medicine, or it could be the result of other factors, including a spontaneous and natural recovery, or the placebo effect. The following criteria were used to choose cases of the highest quality:

- All cases where improvement in both the primary clinical symptom and overall health was recorded within 7 days of commencing homeopathic treatment (ORIDL +3 or + 4) were included, as this is taken to be an indication of the efficacy of the homeopathic remedy.

- Improvements were already noticeable just a few hours after starting homeopathic medication. The treatment period was considered to be twenty-four hours.

- Persistent improvement following multiple administrations of the treatment of choice.

Once all of the relevant information had been entered into the spreadsheet, each of the aforementioned cases was analyzed in greater depth utilizing specific areas of the Modified Naranjo Criteria for determining causal attribution of clinical outcomes [62]. Only the following four of ten possible domains were taken into account.

- Domain 1: Did the primary ailment for which the homeopathic remedy was prescribed improve?

- Domain 2: How quickly did the patient's condition improve after starting treatment?

- Domain 5: Did people feel better overall?

- Domain 10: To what extent does repeated dosage improve clinical outcomes?

In 258 cases, only one homeopathic remedy was provided, whereas in the remaining 69 cases, two or more homeopathic remedies were prescribed in sequence. When RT-PCR testing was performed 2–3 weeks after homeopathic treatment, all 35 instances tested negative. Due to the revised guidelines, testing was not possible in other cases where the patient was discharged after 10 days of symptom onset and no fever for 3 days (in mild cases) or after 10 days of symptom onset and no fever

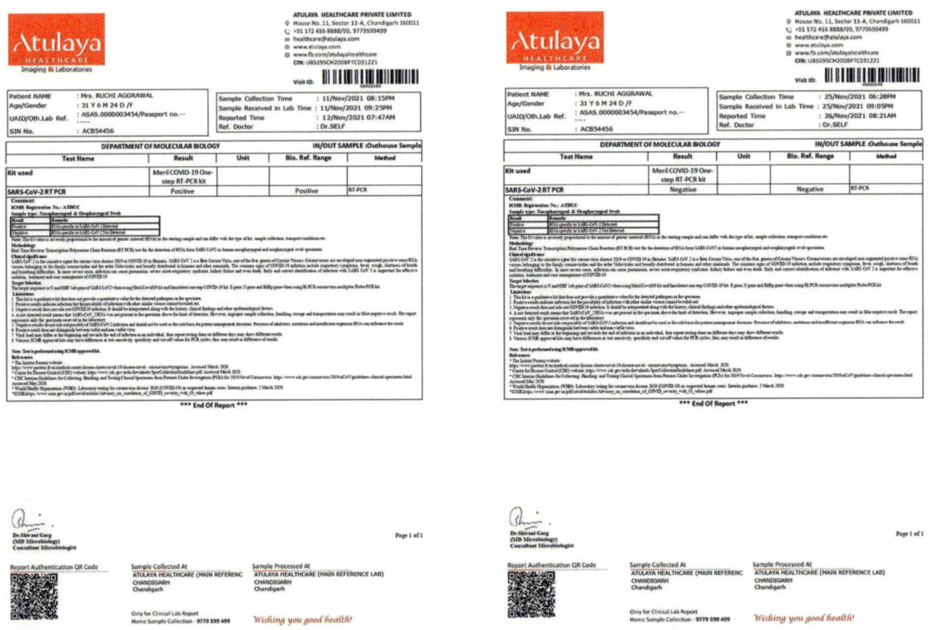

Figure 1.
COVID-19 pre-medication and post medication reports of patient I.

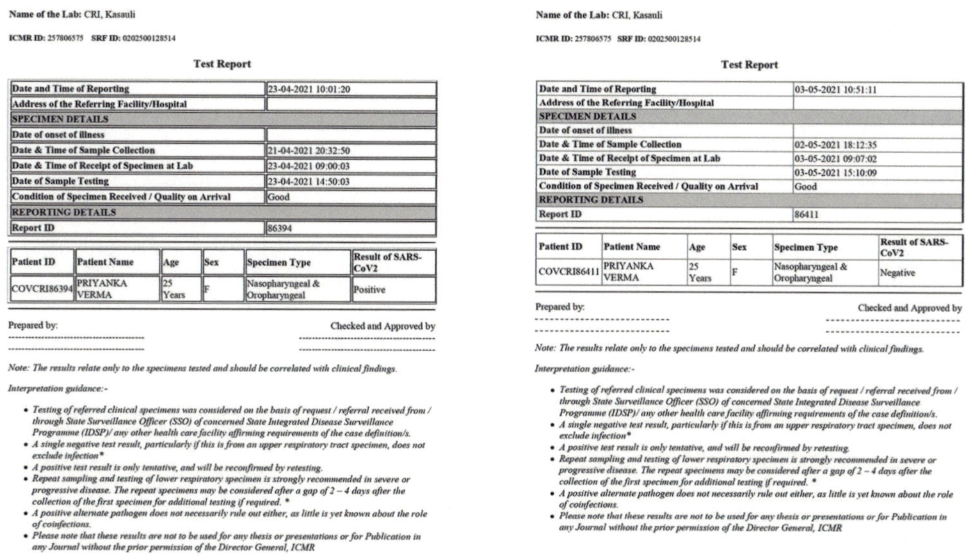

Name of the Lab: CRI, Kasauli

ICMR ID: 257806575 SRF ID: 0202500128514

Test Report

Date and Time of Reporting	23-04-2021 10:01:20
Address of the Referring Facility/Hospital	
SPECIMEN DETAILS	
Date of onset of illness	
Date & Time of Sample Collection	21-04-2021 20:32:50
Date & Time of Receipt of Specimen at Lab	23-04-2021 09:00:03
Date of Sample Testing	23-04-2021 14:50:03
Condition of Specimen Received / Quality on Arrival	Good
REPORTING DETAILS	
Report ID	86394

Patient ID	Patient Name	Age	Sex	Specimen Type	Result of SARS-CoV2
COVCRI86394	PRIYANKA VERMA	25 Years	F	Nasopharyngeal & Oropharyngeal	Positive

Prepared by: Checked and Approved by

Note: The results relate only to the specimens tested and should be correlated with clinical findings.

Interpretation guidance:-

- *Testing of referred clinical specimens was considered on the basis of request / referral received from / through State Surveillance Officer (SSO) of concerned State Integrated Disease Surveillance Programme (IDSP)/ any other health care facility affirming requirements of the case definition/s.*
- *A single negative test result, particularly if this is from an upper respiratory tract specimen, does not exclude infection**
- *A positive test result is only tentative, and will be reconfirmed by retesting.*
- *Repeat sampling and testing of lower respiratory specimen is strongly recommended in severe or progressive disease. The repeat specimens may be considered after a gap of 2 – 4 days after the collection of the first specimen for additional testing if required. **
- *A positive alternate pathogen does not necessarily rule out either, as little is yet known about the role of coinfections.*
- *Please note that these results are not to be used for any thesis or presentations or for Publication in any Journal without the prior permission of the Director General, ICMR*

Name of the Lab: CRI, Kasauli

ICMR ID: 257806575 SRF ID: 0202500128514

Test Report

Date and Time of Reporting	03-05-2021 10:51:11
Address of the Referring Facility/Hospital	
SPECIMEN DETAILS	
Date of onset of illness	
Date & Time of Sample Collection	02-05-2021 18:12:35
Date & Time of Receipt of Specimen at Lab	03-05-2021 09:07:02
Date of Sample Testing	03-05-2021 15:10:09
Condition of Specimen Received / Quality on Arrival	Good
REPORTING DETAILS	
Report ID	86411

Patient ID	Patient Name	Age	Sex	Specimen Type	Result of SARS-CoV2
COVCRI86411	PRIYANKA VERMA	25 Years	F	Nasopharyngeal & Oropharyngeal	Negative

Prepared by: Checked and Approved by

Note: The results relate only to the specimens tested and should be correlated with clinical findings.

Interpretation guidance:-

- *Testing of referred clinical specimens was considered on the basis of request / referral received from / through State Surveillance Officer (SSO) of concerned State Integrated Disease Surveillance Programme (IDSP)/ any other health care facility affirming requirements of the case definition/s.*
- *A single negative test result, particularly if this is from an upper respiratory tract specimen, does not exclude infection**
- *A positive test result is only tentative, and will be reconfirmed by retesting.*
- *Repeat sampling and testing of lower respiratory specimen is strongly recommended in severe or progressive disease. The repeat specimens may be considered after a gap of 2 – 4 days after the collection of the first specimen for additional testing if required. **
- *A positive alternate pathogen does not necessarily rule out either, as little is yet known about the role of coinfections.*
- *Please note that these results are not to be used for any thesis or presentations or for Publication in any Journal without the prior permission of the Director General, ICMR*

Figure 2.
COVID-19 pre-medication and post medication reports of patient II.

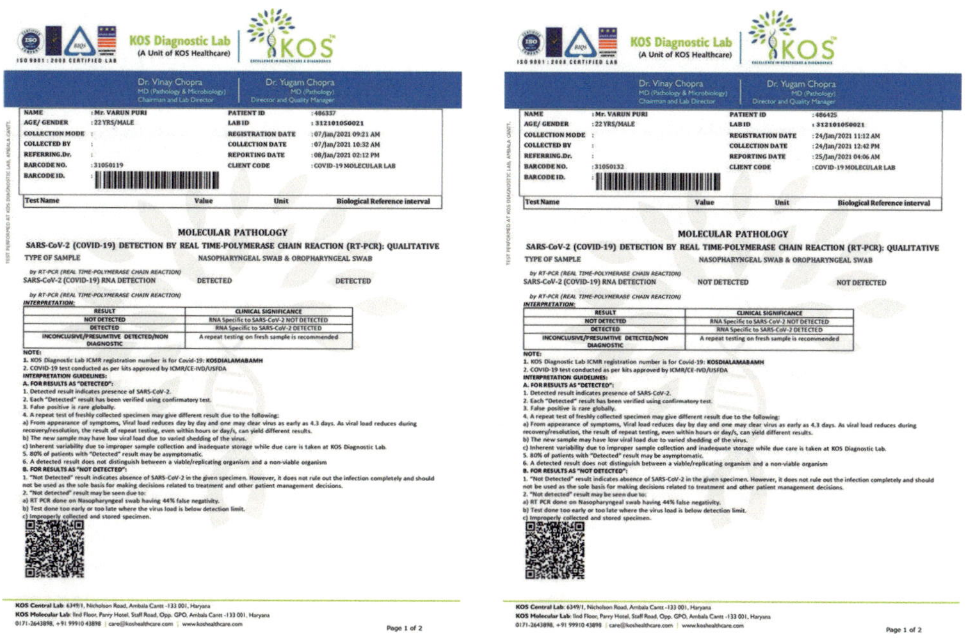

ISO 9001 : 2008 CERTIFIED LAB
KOS Diagnostic Lab
(A Unit of KOS Healthcare)
KOS

Dr. Vinay Chopra
MD (Pathology & Microbiology)
Chairman and Lab Director

Dr. Yugam Chopra
MD (Pathology)
Director and Quality Manager

NAME	: Mr. VARUN PURI	PATIENT ID	: 486337
AGE/ GENDER	: 22 YRS/MALE	LAB ID	: 312101050021
COLLECTION MODE	:	REGISTRATION DATE	: 07/Jan/2021 09:21 AM
COLLECTED BY	:	COLLECTION DATE	: 07/Jan/2021 10:32 AM
REFERRING.Dr.	:	REPORTING DATE	: 08/Jan/2021 02:12 PM
BARCODE NO.	: 31050119	CLIENT CODE	: COVID-19 MOLECULAR LAB
BARCODE ID.	:		

Test Name	Value	Unit	Biological Reference interval

MOLECULAR PATHOLOGY

SARS-CoV-2 (COVID-19) DETECTION BY REAL TIME-POLYMERASE CHAIN REACTION (RT-PCR): QUALITATIVE

TYPE OF SAMPLE NASOPHARYNGEAL SWAB & OROPHARYNGEAL SWAB

by RT-PCR (REAL TIME-POLYMERASE CHAIN REACTION)
SARS-CoV-2 (COVID-19) RNA DETECTION DETECTED DETECTED

by RT-PCR (REAL TIME-POLYMERASE CHAIN REACTION)
INTERPRETATION:

RESULT	CLINICAL SIGNIFICANCE
NOT DETECTED	RNA Specific to SARS-CoV-2 NOT DETECTED
DETECTED	RNA Specific to SARS-CoV-2 DETECTED
INCONCLUSIVE/PRESUMTIVE DETECTED/NON DIAGNOSTIC	A repeat testing on fresh sample is recommended

NOTE:
1. KOS Diagnostic Lab ICMR registration number is for Covid-19: **KOSDIALAMABAMH**
2. COVID-19 test conducted as per kits approved by ICMR/CE-IVD/USFDA

INTERPRETATION GUIDELINES:
A. FOR RESULTS AS "DETECTED":
1. Detected result indicates presence of SARS-CoV-2.
2. Each "Detected" result has been verified using confirmatory test.
3. False positive is rare globally.
4. A repeat test of freshly collected specimen may give different result due to the following:
a) From appearance of symptoms, Viral load reduces day by day and one may clear virus as early as 4.3 days. As viral load reduces during recovery/resolution, the result of repeat testing, even within hours or day/s, can yield different results.
b) The new sample may have low viral load due to varied shedding of the virus.
c) Inherent variability due to improper sample collection and inadequate storage while due care is taken at KOS Diagnostic Lab.
5. 80% of patients with "Detected" result may be asymptomatic.
6. A detected result does not distinguish between a viable/replicating organism and a non-viable organism
B. FOR RESULTS AS "NOT DETECTED":
1. "Not Detected" result indicates absence of SARS-CoV-2 in the given specimen. However, it does not rule out the infection completely and should not be used as the sole basis for making decisions related to treatment and other patient management decisions.
2. "Not detected" result may be seen due to:
a) RT PCR done on Nasopharyngeal swab having 44% false negativity.
b) Test done too early or too late where the virus load is below detection limit.
c) Improperly collected and stored specimen.

KOS Central Lab: 6349/1, Nicholson Road, Ambala Cantt -133 001, Haryana
KOS Molecular Lab: IInd Floor, Parry Hotel, Staff Road, Opp. GPO, Ambala Cantt -133 001, Haryana
0171-2643898, +91 99910 43898 | care@koshealthcare.com | www.koshealthcare.com
Page 1 of 2

ISO 9001 : 2008 CERTIFIED LAB
KOS Diagnostic Lab
(A Unit of KOS Healthcare)
KOS

Dr. Vinay Chopra
MD (Pathology & Microbiology)
Chairman and Lab Director

Dr. Yugam Chopra
MD (Pathology)
Director and Quality Manager

NAME	: Mr. VARUN PURI	PATIENT ID	: 486425
AGE/ GENDER	: 22 YRS/MALE	LAB ID	: 312101050021
COLLECTION MODE	:	REGISTRATION DATE	: 24/Jan/2021 11:12 AM
COLLECTED BY	:	COLLECTION DATE	: 24/Jan/2021 12:42 PM
REFERRING.Dr.	:	REPORTING DATE	: 25/Jan/2021 04:06 AM
BARCODE NO.	: 31050132	CLIENT CODE	: COVID-19 MOLECULAR LAB
BARCODE ID.	:		

Test Name	Value	Unit	Biological Reference interval

MOLECULAR PATHOLOGY

SARS-CoV-2 (COVID-19) DETECTION BY REAL TIME-POLYMERASE CHAIN REACTION (RT-PCR): QUALITATIVE

TYPE OF SAMPLE NASOPHARYNGEAL SWAB & OROPHARYNGEAL SWAB

by RT-PCR (REAL TIME-POLYMERASE CHAIN REACTION)
SARS-CoV-2 (COVID-19) RNA DETECTION NOT DETECTED NOT DETECTED

by RT-PCR (REAL TIME-POLYMERASE CHAIN REACTION)
INTERPRETATION:

RESULT	CLINICAL SIGNIFICANCE
NOT DETECTED	RNA Specific to SARS-CoV-2 NOT DETECTED
DETECTED	RNA Specific to SARS-CoV-2 DETECTED
INCONCLUSIVE/PRESUMTIVE DETECTED/NON DIAGNOSTIC	A repeat testing on fresh sample is recommended

NOTE:
1. KOS Diagnostic Lab ICMR registration number is for Covid-19: **KOSDIALAMABAMH**
2. COVID-19 test conducted as per kits approved by ICMR/CE-IVD/USFDA

INTERPRETATION GUIDELINES:
A. FOR RESULTS AS "DETECTED":
1. Detected result indicates presence of SARS-CoV-2.
2. Each "Detected" result has been verified using confirmatory test.
3. False positive is rare globally.
4. A repeat test of freshly collected specimen may give different result due to the following:
a) From appearance of symptoms, Viral load reduces day by day and one may clear virus as early as 4.3 days. As viral load reduces during recovery/resolution, the result of repeat testing, even within hours or day/s, can yield different results.
b) The new sample may have low viral load due to varied shedding of the virus.
c) Inherent variability due to improper sample collection and inadequate storage while due care is taken at KOS Diagnostic Lab.
5. 80% of patients with "Detected" result may be asymptomatic.
6. A detected result does not distinguish between a viable/replicating organism and a non-viable organism
B. FOR RESULTS AS "NOT DETECTED":
1. "Not Detected" result indicates absence of SARS-CoV-2 in the given specimen. However, it does not rule out the infection completely and should not be used as the sole basis for making decisions related to treatment and other patient management decisions.
2. "Not detected" result may be seen due to:
a) RT PCR done on Nasopharyngeal swab having 44% false negativity.
b) Test done too early or too late where the virus load is below detection limit.
c) Improperly collected and stored specimen.

KOS Central Lab: 6349/1, Nicholson Road, Ambala Cantt -133 001, Haryana
KOS Molecular Lab: IInd Floor, Parry Hotel, Staff Road, Opp. GPO, Ambala Cantt -133 001, Haryana
0171-2643898, +91 99910 43898 | care@koshealthcare.com | www.koshealthcare.com
Page 1 of 2

Figure 3.
COVID-19 pre-medication and post medication reports of patient III.

without antipyretics, resolution of breathlessness, and no oxygen requirement (in moderate cases) [63].

Totaling 211 patients, all of whom showed significant symptom improvement on the COVID-19 scale, were included in the analysis. Insufficient follow-up (22 instances), absence of symptoms (7 cases), and inability to prove causality (42 cases) were among the reasons a total of 116 cases had to be left out of the analysis.

Fatigue, sore throat, dry cough, myalgia, fever, dry mouth and throat, increased thirst, headache, diminished appetite, anxiety, and altered taste were the most often reported side effects. With reference to the above said number of cases, few of them were discussed. The pre COVID and post COVID RT-PCR reports were taken from the patient as shown in **Figures 1–3**. The post COVID reports of three patients (Patient I, II & III) clearly indicates the therapeutic effect of homeopathic remedies which was prescribed by the physician.

These three patients wanted homeopathic treatment in addition to conventional medicine for Integrative Complementary Medicine, and one of them was hospitalized due to moderate to severe COVID-19-related symptoms. Patients I, II, and III were all adults with proven COVID-19 infection upon admission. According to **Table 1** and **Figures 4–6**, they have received their homeopathic drugs from a licensed pharmacy or registered practitioner in the form of a potency and mother tincture (liquid).

Day	Current condition	Homeopathic remedies
Patient I		
1	Heaviness in the right leg; stitching pain on the left of the chest; restlessness; anxiety; weakness and feeling thirsty	*Arsenicum Album* for every 2 hours
2	No fever; no pain around heart	*Arsenicum Album* for every 2 hours
3	No fever, required less supplementary oxygen: walk easly	*Arsenicum Album* for every 2 hours
4	Headache, stable respiratory condition	*Arsenicum Album* for every 2 hours
5	Frontal sinus headache; viscid coryza and tightly adhering scabs in nose	*Arsenicum Album* for every 2 hours; *Kali Bichromicum* for every 4 hours
6	Less headache; feeling better	—
7–14	Hospitalized; Under observation without homeopathic treatments	
14	Patient discharged	
Patient II		
1	Pneumonia; severe thirst for large quantities of cold water; nausea; weakness during fever; drowsiness – constant desire to close eyes; chest pain; alternating chills and sweats; perspiration down back and numbness in legs	*Phosphorus* for every 2 hours
2	Gastrointestinal (GI) symptoms improved; dyspnea; drink greater quantities without feeling nauseous; respiratory symptoms improved; reduced chest pain; hollowness in the chest; weakness during fever	*Arsenicum Album* for every 2 hours; *Phosphoric Acid* for every 2 hours
3	Anxiety and restlessness; cold drinks aggravate; warm ameliorate	*Phosphoric Acid* for every 2 hours; *Stannum* for every 2 hours (alternative)
4	**Homeopathic treatment protocol continued unchanged**	
5	Respiratory symptoms concomitant with abdominal complaints;	*Phosphoric Acid* for every 2 hours; *Bryonia Alba* (Single dose)
6	Patient discharged	

DOI: http://dx.doi.org/10.5772/intechopen.107448

Day	Current condition	Homeopathic remedies
Patient III		
1	Polydipsia; diarrhea; oxygen saturation falling to 87%	*Phosphorus* for every 2 hours
2	Diarrhea stopped; fever normalized; no respiratory improvement	*Phosphorus* for every 2 hours
3	Dyspnea and cough; aggravated by speaking; deep inhalation or prone position; dizzy headache between eyebrows; inability to keep eyes open; chill without shivering' white and paralyzed tongue	*Lobelia Purpurascens* for every 2 hours
4	**Two-hourly** *Lobelia purpurascens* **was continued**	
5	**Two-hourly** *Lobelia purpurascens* **was continued**	
6	Sensation of inhaling smoke and dryness, bifurcation of bronchial tubes which causes coughing	*Ozone* for every 2 hours
7–9	**Ozone 3 times a day**	
10	Patient discharged	

Table 1.
Day wise treatment of patients showed improvement in their health after administration of homeopathic remedies.

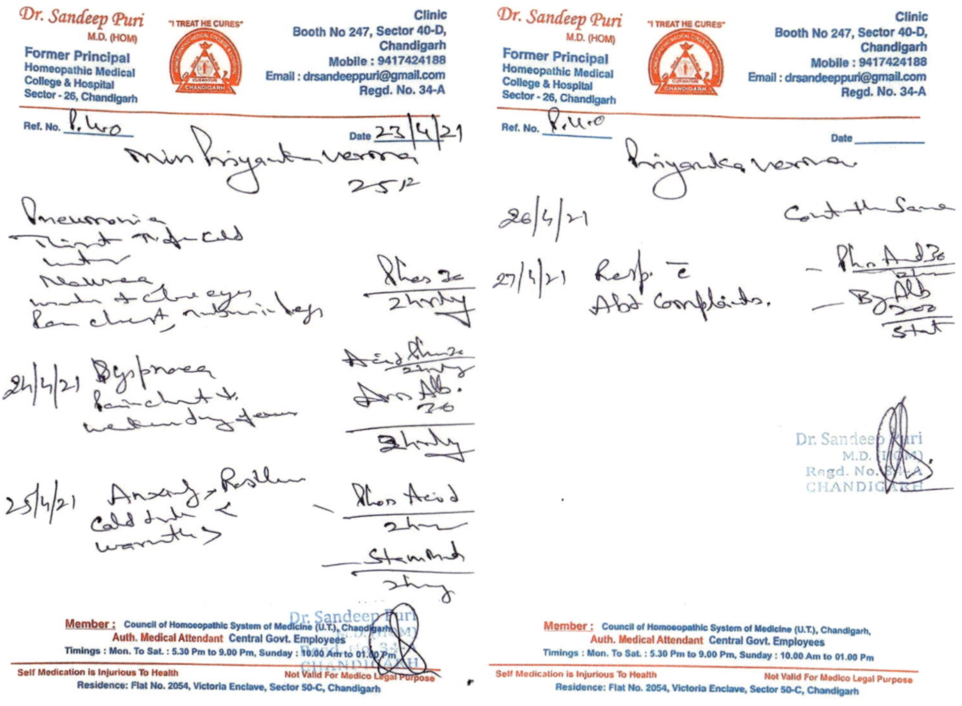
Dr. Sandeep Puri
M.D. (HOM)
Former Principal
Homeopathic Medical College & Hospital
Sector - 26, Chandigarh
"I TREAT HE CURES"
Clinic
Booth No 247, Sector 40-D, Chandigarh
Mobile : 9417424188
Email : drsandeeppuri@gmail.com
Regd. No. 34-A
Ref. No. Date 23/4/21
Mrs Priyanka Verma
Pneumonia
24/4/21 Dyspnoea
25/4/21 Anxiety, Restless
Phos Acid
Member : Council of Homoeopathic System of Medicine (U.T.), Chandigarh,
Auth. Medical Attendant Central Govt. Employees
Timings : Mon. To Sat. : 5.30 Pm to 9.00 Pm, Sunday : 10.00 Am to 01.00 Pm
Self Medication is Injurious To Health Not Valid For Medico Legal Purpose
Residence: Flat No. 2054, Victoria Enclave, Sector 50-C, Chandigarh

Dr. Sandeep Puri
M.D. (HOM)
Former Principal
Homeopathic Medical College & Hospital
Sector - 26, Chandigarh
"I TREAT HE CURES"
Clinic
Booth No 247, Sector 40-D, Chandigarh
Mobile : 9417424188
Email : drsandeeppuri@gmail.com
Regd. No. 34-A
Ref. No. Date
Priyanka Verma
26/4/21 Cont the Same
27/4/21 Resp. Abd Complaints.
Dr. Sandeep Puri
M.D. (HOM)
Regd. No. 34-A
CHANDIGARH
Member : Council of Homoeopathic System of Medicine (U.T.), Chandigarh,
Auth. Medical Attendant Central Govt. Employees
Timings : Mon. To Sat. : 5.30 Pm to 9.00 Pm, Sunday : 10.00 Am to 01.00 Pm
Self Medication is Injurious To Health Not Valid For Medico Legal Purpose
Residence: Flat No. 2054, Victoria Enclave, Sector 50-C, Chandigarh

Figure 4.
Prescription of patient-I received from a registered practitioner or physician.

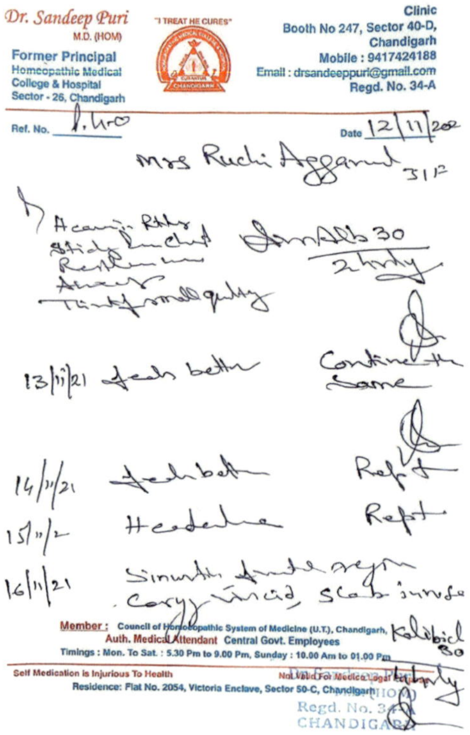
Dr. Sandeep Puri
M.D. (HOM)
"I TREAT HE CURES"
Former Principal
Homeopathic Medical College & Hospital
Sector - 26, Chandigarh
Clinic
Booth No 247, Sector 40-D, Chandigarh
Mobile : 9417424188
Email : drsandeeppuri@gmail.com
Regd. No. 34-A
Ref. No.
Date 12/11/202
Mrs Ruchi Aggarwal 31 F
13/11/21 feels better — Continue the same
14/11/21 — Repeat
15/11/2 Headache — Repeat
16/11/21
Member : Council of Homoeopathic System of Medicine (U.T.), Chandigarh,
Auth. Medical Attendant Central Govt. Employees
Timings : Mon. To Sat. : 5.30 Pm to 9.00 Pm, Sunday : 10.00 Am to 01.00 Pm
Self Medication is Injurious To Health
Not Valid For Medico Legal Purpose
Residence: Flat No. 2054, Victoria Enclave, Sector 50-C, Chandigarh

Figure 5.
Prescription of patient-II received from a registered practitioner or physician.

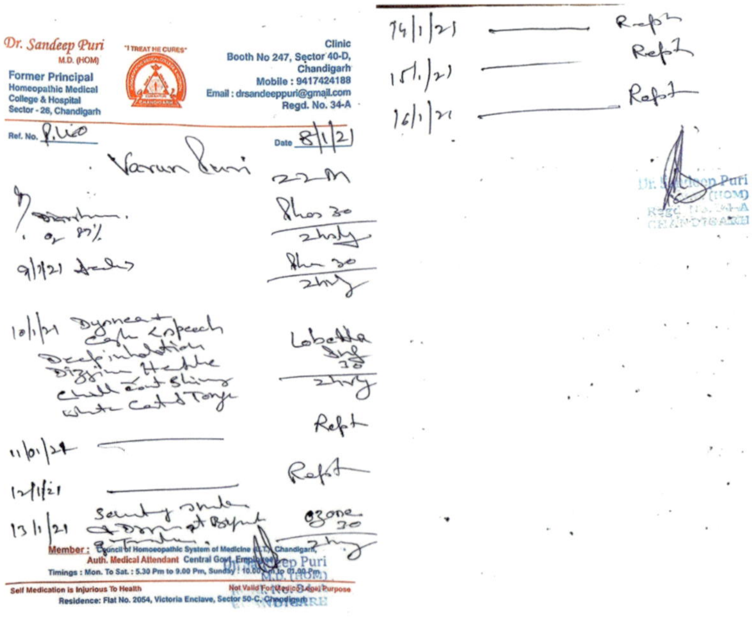
Dr. Sandeep Puri
M.D. (HOM)
"I TREAT HE CURES"
Former Principal
Homeopathic Medical College & Hospital
Sector - 26, Chandigarh
Clinic
Booth No 247, Sector 40-D, Chandigarh
Mobile : 9417424188
Email : drsandeeppuri@gmail.com
Regd. No. 34-A
Ref. No.
Date 8/1/21
Varun Puri 22 M
9/1/21
10/1/21
11/01/21 — Repeat
12/1/21 — Repeat
13/1/21
14/1/21 — Repeat
15/1/21 — Repeat
16/1/21 — Repeat
Member : Council of Homoeopathic System of Medicine (U.T.), Chandigarh,
Auth. Medical Attendant Central Govt. Employees
Timings : Mon. To Sat. : 5.30 Pm to 9.00 Pm, Sunday : 10.00 Am to 01.00 Pm
Self Medication is Injurious To Health
Not Valid For Medico Legal Purpose
Residence: Flat No. 2054, Victoria Enclave, Sector 50-C, Chandigarh

Figure 6.
Prescription of patient-III received from a registered practitioner or physician.

6. Conclusions

The symptoms of COVID-19 patients were said to have improved due to homeopathic treatments. Findings from case studies can help with homeopathic prescribing in future controlled research on COVID-19. Most of the symptoms of this pandemic can be helped by homeopathic treatment, which adds to the medications domain of action. In addition, it has been demonstrated that homeopathic medicines can alleviate symptoms across the spectrum of the diseases manifestations. Supportive evidence suggests that homeopathic treatments could be used alongside conventional preventative and curative methods during the current COVID-19 outbreak.

Acknowledgements

The authors would like to express their gratitude to Dr. Madhu Chitkara, Vice-Chancellor of Chitkara University, Punjab, India; Dr. Ashok Chitkara, Chancellor of Chitkara University, Punjab, India; and Dr. Nitin Verma, Principal of the School of Pharmacy at Chitkara University, Himachal Pradesh, India.

Conflict of interest

The authors declare no conflict of interest.

Author details

Ameya Sharma[1], Sandeep Puri[2], Varun Puri[2], Divya Dheer[1], Neha Bhandari[1] and Vivek Puri[1*]

1 Chitkara School of Pharmacy, Chitkara University, Himachal Pradesh, India

2 Homoeopathic Medical College and Hospital, Chandigarh, India

*Address all correspondence to: vivek.puri@chitkara.edu.in

References

[1] Riou J, Althaus CL. Pattern of early human-to-human transmission of Wuhan 2019 novel coronavirus (2019-nCoV), December 2019 to January 2020. Eurosurveillance. 2020;**25**(4):2000058

[2] Zhang H, Chen Y, Yuan Q, Xia QX, Zeng XP, Peng JT, et al. Identification of kidney transplant recipients with coronavirus disease 2019. European Urology. 2020;**77**(6):742-747

[3] Coronavirus: The first three months as it happened. Available from: https://www.nature.com/articles/d41586-020-00154-w

[4] Huang C, Wang Y, Li X, Ren L, Zhao J, Hu Y, et al. Clinical features of patients infected with 2019 novel coronavirus in Wuhan, China. The Lancet. 2020;**395**(10223):497-506

[5] Ghebrehiwet B, Peerschke EI. Complement and coagulation: Key triggers of COVID-19–induced multiorgan pathology. The Journal of Clinical Investigation. 2020;**130**(11):5674-5676

[6] Chen N, Zhou M, Dong X, Qu J, Gong F, Han Y, et al. Epidemiological and clinical characteristics of 99 cases of 2019 novel coronavirus pneumonia in Wuhan, China: A descriptive study. The Lancet. 2020;**395**(10223):507-513

[7] Thierry AR, Roch B. SARS-CoV2 may evade innate immune response, causing uncontrolled neutrophil extracellular traps formation and multi-organ failure. Clinical Science. 2020;**134**(12):1295-1300

[8] Zhu RF, Gao YL, Robert SH, Gao JP, Yang SG, Zhu CT. Systematic review of the registered clinical trials for coronavirus disease 2019 (COVID-19). Journal of Translational Medicine. 2020;**18**(1):1-9

[9] Zhou H, Fang Y, Xu T, Ni WJ, Shen AZ, Meng XM. Potential therapeutic targets and promising drugs for combating SARS-CoV-2. British Journal of Pharmacology. 2020;**177**(14):3147-3161

[10] Brant AC, Tian W, Majerciak V, Yang W, Zheng ZM. SARS-CoV-2: From its discovery to genome structure, transcription, and replication. Cell & Bioscience. 2021;**11**(1):1-7

[11] Cheng L, Zhang X, Chen Y, Wang D, Zhang D, Yan S, et al. Dynamic landscape mapping of humoral immunity to SARS-CoV-2 identifies non-structural protein antibodies associated with the survival of critical COVID-19 patients. Signal Transduction and Targeted Therapy. 2021;**6**(1):1-4

[12] Littler DR, Gully BS, Colson RN, Rossjohn J. Crystal structure of the SARS-CoV-2 non-structural protein 9, Nsp9. Iscience. 2020;**23**(7):101258

[13] Golovkin A, Kalinina O, Bezrukikh V, Aquino A, Zaikova E, Karonova T, et al. Imbalanced immune response of T-cell and B-cell subsets in patients with moderate and severe COVID-19. Viruses. 2021;**13**(10):1966

[14] WHO recommends highly successful COVID-19 therapy and calls for wide geographical distribution and transparency from originator. Available from: https://www.who.int/news/item/22-04-2022-who-recommends-highly-successful-covid-19-therapy-and-calls-for-wide-geographical-distribution-and-transparency-from-originator

[15] Safety issues in the preparation of homeopathic medicines. Available from: https://apps.who.int/iris/bitstream/

handle/10665/44238/9789241598842_eng.pdf

[16] Homeopathic Products. Available from: https://www.fda.gov/drugs/information-drug-class/homeopathic-products

[17] Bellavite P, Chirumbolo S, Magnani P, Ortolani R, Conforti A. Effectiveness of homeopathy in immunology and inflammation disorders. A literature overview of clinical studies. Homoeopathic Heritage International. 2008;**33**(2):35-37

[18] Kent JT. Lectures on Homoeopathic Philosophy. New Delhi: Jain Publishers; 1993. pp. 92-93

[19] Takacs M, Frass M, Walder G, Fibert P, Rottensteiner M, Glück W, et al. Adjunctive homeopathic treatment of hospitalized COVID-19 patients (COVIHOM): A retrospective case series. Complementary Therapies in Clinical Practice. 2021;**44**:101415

[20] Hahnemann S. Organon of Medicine. 6th ed. New Delhi: Jain Publishers; 1994

[21] Swayne J. International Dictionary of Homeopathy. Edinburgh, London: Churchill Livingstone; 2000. p. 222

[22] Linde K, Clausius N, Ramirez G, Melchart D, Eitel F, Hedges LV, et al. Are the clinical effects of homoeopathy placebo effects? A meta-analysis of placebo-controlled trials. The Lancet. 1997;**350**(9081):834-843

[23] Srikanth N, Rana RK, Jameela S, Singhal R, Tripathi A, Khanduri S, et al. Perception and practices followed by AYUSH practitioners and health seekers for prevention of COVID-19: Cross-sectional analysis of an app-based data. OSF Preprints. 2021. DOI:10.31219/osf.io/b6jqv

[24] Jethani B, Gupta M, Wadhwani P, Thomas R, Balakrishnan T, Mathew G, et al. Clinical characteristics and remedy profiles of patients with COVID-19: A retrospective cohort study. Homeopathy. 2021;**110**(02):086-093

[25] Azis SP, Kaur H. Enabling use of homoeopathy in India's preparedness for pandemic/epidemic situation like COVID-19. Indian Journal of Research in Homoeopathy. 2020;**14**(2):143

[26] Chaudhary A, Khurana A. A review on the role of homoeopathy in epidemics with some reflections on COVID-19 (SARS-CoV-2). Indian Journal of Research in Homoeopathy. 2020;**14**(2):100

[27] Goswami S, Dey C. Role of Homoeopathy in Prophylaxis and the Symptomatic management of influenza-Like Illnesses (COVID-19) Patients. In COVID-19 and SARS-CoV-2. Boca Raton: CRC Press; 2022. pp. 219-228

[28] Manchanda RK, Miglani A, Gupta M, Meena BS, Chadha V, Joseph F, et al. Homeopathic remedies in COVID-19: Prognostic factor research. Homeopathy. 2021;**110**(03):160-167

[29] Parikh N, Parikh D, Parikh D. Role of homoeopathy in COVID-19 management—A clinical experience. World Journal of Pharmaceutical Research. 2020;**9**(5):2459

[30] Cascella M, Rajnik M, Aleem A, Dulebohn SC, Di Napoli R. Features, Evaluation, and Treatment of Coronavirus (COVID-19). 2022. StatPearls [Internet]. PMID: 32150360

[31] Coronavirus Disease 2019 (COVID-19): Testing for COVID-19. Centers for Disease Control and Prevention. Available from: https://www.cdc.gov/coronavirus/2019-ncov/symptoms-testing/testing.html. [Accessed: April 13, 2020]

[32] Hasan N, Nayem MU, Mohshinuzzaman M, Biswas AH, Kayes ME, Hakim MA, et al. Homeopathic approach to COVID-19: A review. Malaysian Journal of Medical and Biological Research. 2020;7(2):81-86

[33] Dasgupta A. Indian Authorities Propose Use of Homeopathy to Prevent Coronavirus [Online]. The Scientist. Available from: https://www.the-scientist.com/news-opinion/indian-authorities-propose-use-of-homeopathy-to-prevent-coronavirus-67075; 2020. [Accessed: April 07, 2020]

[34] Najima Parveen D, Rasheed B, Vishnoi NK, Ajitha Rani D, Bharadwaj A, Singh P. Homoeopathic approach in COVID-19 pandemic condition: A review. International Journal of Homoeopathic Sciences. 2021;**5**(3):77-78

[35] Gupta P, Sundaram EN, Sharma M, Prajapati S, Arya BS, Khurana A, et al. Pre-clinical pharmacology: An important aspect in homoeopathic research. 2018. Available from: http://aohindia.in:8080/xmlui/handle/123456789/1852

[36] Singh RS, Singh A, Kaur H, Batra G, Sarma P, Kaur H, et al. Promising traditional Indian medicinal plants for the management of novel coronavirus disease: A systematic review. Phytotherapy Research. 2021;**35**(8):4456-4484

[37] Pal PP, Ningthoujam G. Research review of genus Epidemicus. International Journal of Advanced Ayurveda, Yoga, Unani, Siddha and Homeopathy. 2019;**8**:545-550

[38] Hahnemann S. Materia Medica Pura. New Delhi: Jain Publishers; 1994

[39] Hahnemann S. Cause and prevention of the asiatic cholera. United States Medical Investigator (1875-1887). 1884;**20**(9):149

[40] Ullman D. Homeopathy-medicine for the 21st-century. Futurist. 1988;**22**(4):43-47

[41] Milgrom LR. Genus epidemicus: Are notions of entanglement relevant to the homeopathic understanding of epidemic disease? Complementary Medicine Research. 2016;**23**(5):290-300

[42] Golden I, Bracho G. A reevaluation of the effectiveness of homoeoprophylaxis against leptospirosis in Cuba in 2007 and 2008. Journal of Evidence-based Complementary & Alternative Medicine. 2014;**19**(3):155-160

[43] Srigiri CG, Muraleedharan KC. A review on coagulopathy in Covid-19 and its Homoeopathic management. International Journal of Homoeopathic Sciences. 2020;**4**(3):369-375

[44] Varanasi R, Nayak D, Khurana A. Clinical repurposing of medicines is intrinsic to homeopathy: Research initiatives on COVID-19 in India. Homeopathy. 2021;**110**(03):198-205

[45] Bhawar P, Bisen P. Psychological problems during COVID-19 and its homoeopathic management. Journal of Medical and Pharmaceutical Innovations. 2021;**8**(44):36-39

[46] Dutta A. Role of homeopathy in epidemics: Paving way for a plausible solution in the management of COVID-19/SARS-CoV-2 infection. Homœopathic Links. 2020;**33**(04):297-301

[47] Adler UC, Adler MS, Padula AE, Hotta LM, de Toledo CA, Diniz JN, et al. Homeopathy for COVID-19 in primary care: A randomized, double-blind, placebo-controlled trial (COVID-simile study). Journal of Integrative Medicine. 2022;**20**(3):221-229

[48] Adler UC, Adler MS, Hotta LM, Padula AE, de Toledo CA, Diniz JN, et al.

Homeopathy for Covid-19 in primary care: A structured summary of a study protocol for a randomized controlled trial. Trials. 2021;**22**(1):1-3

[49] Savera KK, Dastagiri P, Muraleedharan KC. Emerging evidence of homoeopathy in treating COVID-19 pandemic: An overview. International Journal of Home Science. 2020;**4**(3):160-166

[50] Mukherjee SK, Ganguly S, Das S, Chatterjee KK, Naskar KK, Dey S, et al. Homeopathic medicines used as prophylaxis in Kolkata during the COVID-19 pandemic: A community-based, cluster-randomized trial. Homeopathy. 2022;**111**(02):097-104

[51] Shinde V, Bawaskar R. Homoeopathy for post COVID 19 illnesses: A case series. Indian Journal of Research in Homoeopathy. 2021;**15**(3):4

[52] Moorthi SK, Radhika P, Muraleedharan KC. Psychological implications during the outbreak of COVID-19 and its homoeopathic management. Indian Journal of Research in Homoeopathy. 2020;**14**(2):136

[53] Rutten L, Miglani A, Gold P, Manchanda RK, Chakraborty M, Meena BS, et al. Generalizability of homeopathic prognostic factor research outcome in COVID-19 treatment: Comparison of data. Homeopathy. Aug 2022;**111**(03):157-163

[54] Islam MA. Role of Lachesis and Gripp heel in the treatment of COVID-19. Homœopathic Links. 2020;**33**(03):233-234

[55] Nambison NK, Nambison SN, Dwivedi AD. Pandemic COVID-19: Homeopathic prevention and treatment experiences. International Journal of Homoeopathic Sciences. 2020;**4**(2): 265-270

[56] Kovilacar R, Misra P. A diagnosed case of COVID-19 treated with homoeopathy: A case report. Homœopathic Links. 2020;**33**(03):241-243

[57] Achner J. Homöopathie als Überlebensstrategie: Stärkung des Immunsystems, Homöopathische Selbstbehandlung, SARS-CoV-2 und Impffolgen. Die Behandlung von Epidemien. BoD–Books on Demand; 2020

[58] Ścibior A, Pietrzyk Ł, Plewa Z, Skiba A. Vanadium: Risks and possible benefits in the light of a comprehensive overview of its pharmacotoxicological mechanisms and multi-applications with a summary of further research trends. Journal of Trace Elements in Medicine and Biology. 2020;**61**:126508

[59] Kleijnen J, Knipschild P, ter Riet G. Clinical trials of homoeopathy. British Medical Journal. 1991;**302**(6772): 316-323

[60] Clinical Management Protocol: COVID-19. Available from: https://www.mohfw.gov.in/pdf/ClinicalManagementProtocolforCOVID19dated27062020.pdf. [Accessed: August 1, 2020]

[61] Reilly D, Mercer SW, Bikker AP, Harrison T. Outcome related to impact on daily living: Preliminary validation of the ORIDL instrument. BMC Health Services Research. 2007;**7**:139

[62] van Haselen RA. Homeopathic clinical case reports: Development of a supplement (HOM-CASE) to the CARE clinical case reporting guideline. Complementary Therapies in Medicine. 2016;**25**:78-85

[63] Revised discharge policy for COVID-19.pdf. Available from: http://health.delhigovt.nic.in/wps/wcm/connect/b6af6e004e9fefb89ce8bd5dc9149193/Order11620.pdf?MOD=AJPERES&lmod=-1471732290&CACHEID=b6af6e004e9fefb89ce8bd5dc9149193. [Accessed: August 1, 2020]

Section 3

Cases Treatment and Management

Chapter 5

Treatments for the Infection by SARS-CoV-2

Nicolás Padilla-Raygoza, Gilberto Flores-Vargas, María de Jesús Gallardo-Luna, Efraín Navarro-Olivos, Francisco Javier Magos-Vázquez and Daniel Alberto Díaz-Martínez

Abstract

In late 2019, pneumonia cases from unknown origin were detected in Wuhan, China. The cause was a new coronavirus. The World Health Organization (WHO) named the virus SARS-CoV-2 and COVID-19 the associated disease. In the first months of 2020, this disease became a pandemic with a high lethality reported. Since then, the search for treatments began. We started by searching among treatments previously approved for human use that were not designed for COVID-19 and were considered to treat this condition. We continued searching on the therapeutics guidelines published by the WHO for the management of infection by SARS-CoV-2. Based on these results, we searched for the literature in PubMed to obtain further evidence on the drugs against SARS-CoV-2. The treatments presented in this chapter are Ivermectin, Hydroxychloroquine, Nitazoxanide, Azithromycin, Molnupiravir, Casirivimab-Imdevimab, Ritonavir-Nirmatrelvir, Ritonavir-Lopinavir, Remdesivir, and Favipiravir. Two years ahead of the start of the COVID-19 pandemic, a plenty of options for treatment have been investigated. Only a few of them have been shown to be efficient and safe. According to the WHO, Ritonavir-Nirmatrelvir outperforms other proposed therapeutics.

Keywords: COVID-19, SARS-CoV-2, therapeutics, molnuparivir, nirmatrelvir

1. Introduction

In late 2019, cases of pneumonia from unknown origin were detected in Wuhan, China. It was concluded that the cause was a new coronavirus [1, 2]. The World Health Organization (WHO) named the virus SARS-CoV-2 and COVID-19 the associated disease [1, 2]. In the first months of 2020, this disease became a pandemic with a reported high lethality. Since then, the search for treatments has begun.

SARS-CoV-2 is a coronavirus of the beta family and is related to the previously known SARS-CoV [3]. It is transmissible from human to human. The primary transmission is via respiratory droplets. Even so, transmission by other fluids has been reported. The protein that mediates the entry to the host cells is the so-called spike protein. It uses the angiotensin-converting enzyme 2 (ACE2) as a cellular receptor. It primarily affects the lungs and the respiratory system with flu-like symptoms presentation [3]. Nevertheless, it also causes a wide spectrum of conditions from diarrhea to loss of smell and taste. The chief complication due to COVID-19 that can lead to death is pneumonia.

Once the SARS-CoV-2 enters the host cell, the viral RNA is attached to the host ribosome, translating into two large coterminal polyproteins. These proteins are then digested into components by proteolysis for packaging new virions. The papain-like protease (PLpro) and the coronavirus main protease (Mpro) are two proteases involved in this process. SARS-CoV-2 employs RNA-dependent RNA polymerase (RdRp) to replicate the genome of RNA. The four proteins: spike, Mpro, PLpro, and RdRp, are essential to virus assembly and pathogenesis. Mpro and RdRp are the targets for drugs against SARS-CoV-2 [4].

This pandemic has disrupted the global society. Besides global health, it has affected the economy and way of living since most of the interventions to stop the dissemination were non-pharmaceutical. Governments around the world exhorted people to stay at home and social distancing [5].

As a result of the global concern posed by this disease, some experiential recommendations emerged for its treatment. Social networks played a crucial role in the diffusion of these recommendations [6]. A couple of cases are hydroxychloroquine and ivermectin [7]. Much of the supposed evidence was absent or anecdotic. It generated false expectations and misinformation.

There were no previously approved therapeutics for COVID-19 since it was an emerging disease. Later in the pandemic, the WHO authorize the emergency use of some antivirals [8, 9]. The recommendations by other institutions of treatments for use outside of clinical trials were scarce. Such is the case for ivermectin [10].

This chapter aims to review the literature on therapeutics approved by the WHO for emergency use. It will also cover some of the treatments recommended and considered based on empirical results.

2. Material and methods

2.1 Search criteria

It was searched on the therapeutics guidelines published by the WHO [11] and the USA Federal Drug Administration (FDA) [12] for the management of infection by SARS-CoV-2. Based on these results, we searched for more literature in PubMed to obtain evidence from the drugs against SARS-CoV-2.

Besides searching for articles in Pubmed, we used the Google Scholar database to search about treatments against SARS-CoV-2 infection, including the words: Treatment, SARS-CoV-2, COVID-19, Therapeutics, WHO approved COVID-19 drugs, and FDA approved COVID-19 drugs.

The chief inclusion criteria were articles on treatments approved by WHO [11] and FDA [12]. The search also included treatments previously approved for human use but not for COVID-19 and, even so, were used.

3. Treatments suggested empirically

There are reports on drugs used empirically for the treatment of COVID-19, and the WHO has made statements on these treatments.

Drug	Indication
Ivermectin	Antiparasitic
Hydroxychloroquine	Antimalarial
Nitazoxanide	Antiparasitic
Azithromycin	Antibiotic

Table 1.
Some drugs used empirically without approval for emergency use.

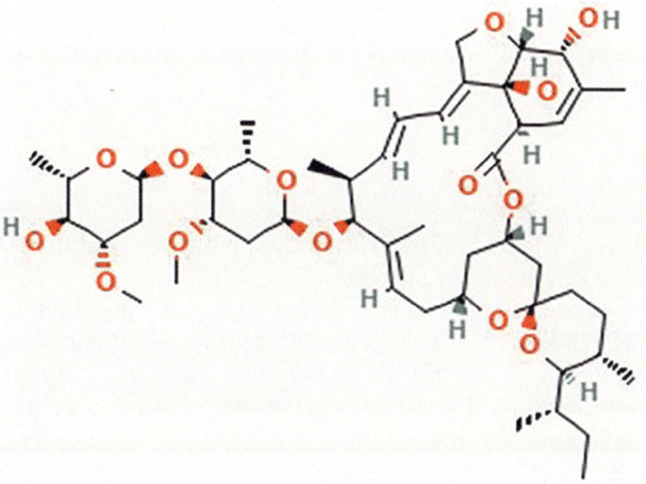

Figure 1.
Chemical structure of ivermectin. Source. Modified from: PubChem. National Library of Medicine [13].

Table 1 shows the drugs of empirical use without approval by the WHO and FDA, for their use against COVID-19 in humans, except in clinical trial settings.

3.1 Ivermectin

Ivermectin is a mixture of 22, 23-dihydroavermectin B1a, and 22, 23-dihydroavermectin B1b. It is macrocyclic lactose with a wide antiparasitic spectrum [10]. Its chemical structure [13], is shown in **Figure 1**.

It is considered that its action mechanism is by inhibiting the nuclear transport mediated by the heterodimer importin α/β1-responsible for the viral protein's translocation (HIV-1, SV40)-, necessary for its replication [14–16]. It has been reported that ivermectin inhibits the SARS-CoV-2 in vitro without stating clearly how it happens [16]. Since then, it was considered a potential treatment.

Even as studies suggest a reduction in mortality, most have methodological deficiencies [17–19]. Hence, further and rigorous evidence on the use of ivermectin against COVID-19 is necessary. Currently, the use of ivermectin is just recommended in clinical trial settings. Also, the Food and Drug Administration does not recommend the ivermectin use against COVID-19 due to the lack of evidence [20]. The same conclusion is supported by the Sanitary Technologies Assess Department from the Clinical and Sanitary Efficacy Institute [21].

The Pan American Health Organization states that there is no certainty about the risks and benefits from the use of ivermectin [22].

3.2 Hydroxychloroquine

Hydroxychloroquine is a 4-aminoquinoline drug aimed to treat malaria and rheumatologic conditions [22]. In **Figure 2**, its chemical structure is shown.

Due to the inhibition of SARS-CoV-2 in vitro, it was considered a potential treatment for COVID-19 [24]. Hydroxychloroquine received much public attention even at high political levels. It caused such a phenomenon that most random trials studying it were unable to finish properly, and those that were completed did not show any benefit [25].

Currently, the WHO makes a strong recommendation against its use in its latest therapeutics guidelines [11, 26].

3.3 Nitazoxanide

Nitazoxanide and its metabolite Tizoxanide could inhibit the in vitro growth of the canine coronavirus S-378 [26]. Wang M et al. [25] have reported that Nitazoxanide could also inhibit the SARS-CoV-2 growth (**Figure 3**).

Early studies suggested a beneficial effect of Nitazoxanide by reducing the disease severity of COVID-19 [28, 29]. Rocco et al [30], reported that Nitazoxanide did not show a difference in preventing admission to the intensive care unit for COVID-19 patients with pneumonia. In this study, it was showed a difference in secondary outcomes such as hospital discharge.

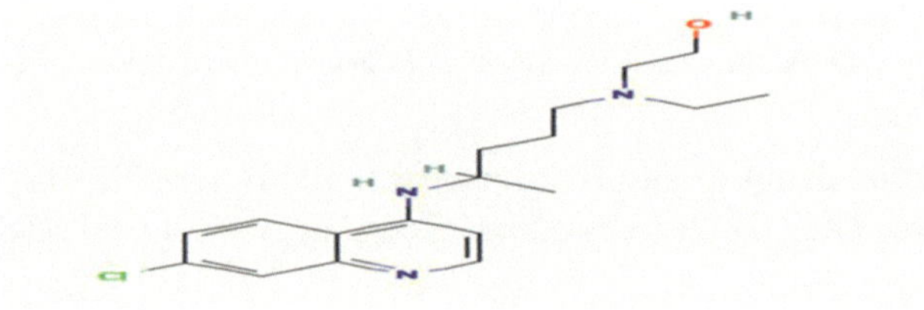

Figure 2.
Chemical structure of hydroxychloroquine. Source: Modified from PubChem. National Library of Medicine [23].

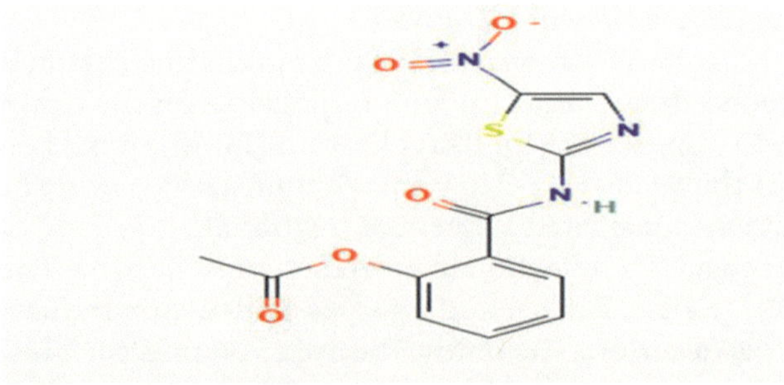

Figure 3.
Chemical structure of Nitazoxanide. Source: Modified from PubChem. National Library of Medicine [27].

There are few studies analyzing Nitazoxanide. So far, there is no evidence of a significant benefit for the COVID-19 treatment. The evidence on the use of nitazoxanide is scarce. The WHO does not include this drug in its living guideline for therapeutics and COVID-19 [11].

3.4 Azithromycin

Azithromycin is an antibiotic mainly prescribed for bacterial diseases and belongs to the family of macrolide [31]. This drug has been considered for COVID-19 treatment due to in vitro results. Its chemical structure is shown in **Figure 4**.

Oldenburg et al. [31], reported the results of a clinical trial involving azithromycin as a candidate. The primary outcome was the resolution of symptoms. It was not found a statistically significant effect between the experimental and the control group. From 23 secondary outcomes, only 5 showed statistically significant differences [33].

Azithromycin was chiefly used with other drugs. As it was used in combination with hydroxychloroquine, its effect and possible harms could not be clearly distinguished [34]. Nevertheless, so far, it is not recommended for COVID-19 treatment. The WHO only includes this drug tangentially in its therapeutics and COVID-19 living guideline while mentioning its use accompanied by hydroxychloroquine [11].

4. Treatments against COVID-19 considered for emergency use

In the following sections, we review some of the therapeutics and their recommendation status by the WHO [11] and FDA [12]. **Table 2** shows the drugs and treatments against COVID-19 treated in this section.

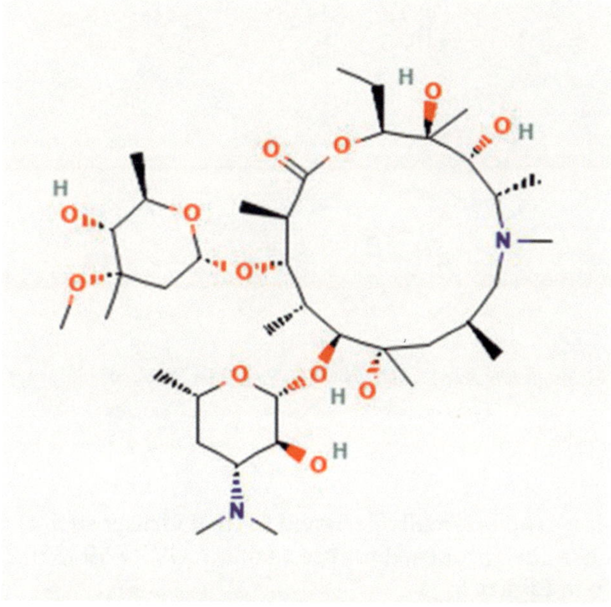

Figure 4.
Chemical structure of azithromycin. Source: Modified from PubChem. National Library of Medicine [32].

Drug	Indication	Dose	Observations
Molnupiravir	For patients with mild COVID-19 with hospitalization risk.	800 mg (four pills) twice a day for 5 days	Do not administer in children or pregnant women. There are no data about its safety.
Casirivimab-Imdevimab	Do not recommend for variants.	Intravenous. Ranging from 1200–2400 mg the total dose	The hospitalization risk decreases by 85%.
Ritonavir-Nirmatrelvir	Recommended as early as possible within the first 5 days since the onset of symptoms.	300 mg (two 150 mg tablets) of nirmatrelvir and 100 mg of ritonavir every 12 hours daily for 5 days	
Remdesivir	Recommended as early as possible within the first 7 days since the onset of symptoms.	Intravenous administration for 3 consecutive days with the following scheme: Day one: 200 mg Day two and three: 100 mg	Conditional recommendation since the existence of potentially most beneficial treatments.
Favipiravir		Not standardized yet	In animal models, it has potentiated the effect of molnupiravir.

Table 2.
Drugs for the emergency use against COVID-19.

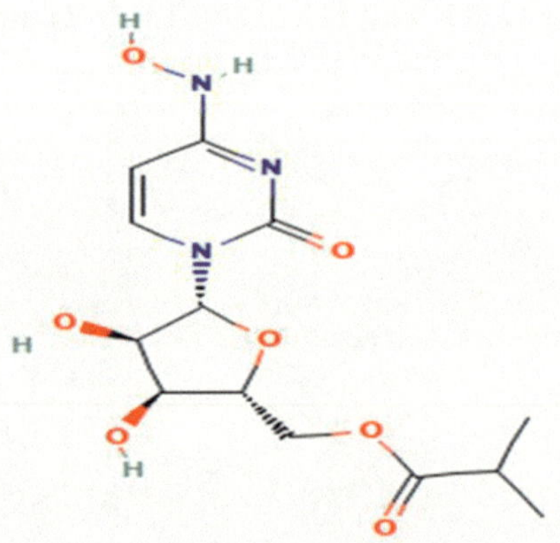

Figure 5.
Chemical structure of Molnupiravir. Source: Modified from PubChem. National Library of Medicine [36].

4.1 Molnupiravir

Molnupiravir is a drug originally designed to treat viruses such as influenza. In recent months, it has been proposed for use against COVID-19 [35]. The chemical structure is shown in **Figure 5**.

In the study by Jayk Bernal et al. [37], the molnupiravir group had better outcomes than the placebo one. The chief outcome was hospitalization or death.

Even as the sex was imbalanced, further analysis showed that the effect remained. There were no statistically significant differences regarding adverse events among the groups.

Singh et al. [35] conclude that the current evidence suggests that molnupiravir is effective for the prevention of hospitalization and deaths in mild COVID-19 patients. Nevertheless, further evidence is needed for the case of moderate and severe COVID-19 patients. Even far, Extance [38], mentions that the existence of only one pivotal study indicates that the evidence is very limited.

The WHO recommends the use of this drug conditionally due to the absence of data about long-term harms that may cause its use [11].

4.2 Casirivimab-Imdevimab

Casirivimab and imdevimab are monoclonal antibodies that target sites in the receptor binding domain of the SARS-CoV-2 spike glycoprotein [39]. The administration via has been one of the chief difficulties for their extensive use—its administration is intravenous.

The RECOVERY Collaboration Group included this treatment in their analysis [39]. They noted that casirivimab-imdevimab reduced the mortality significatively among seronegative patients (those without previously mounted humoral response).

The WHO recommends it conditionally. The reasons are that other drugs have proven to be more effective and safer. Also, these drugs are easiest to administer [11].

4.3 Ritonavir-Nirmatrelvir

Nirmatrelvir is a drug designed to treat covid-19 by targeting its main protease [40]. It has been administered with ritonavir. **Figure 6** shows the chemical structure of nirmatrelvir and ritonavir.

Hammond et al. [40] report that the incidence of hospitalization or death was lower by approximately 6% points in the treatment group than in the control group—observed in the interim and final analysis. The difference among adverse events was not statistically significant.

Its first approval for conditional use was issued in the United Kingdom on December 31, 2021. Since then, other countries have approved this drug in different modalities, such as for emergency use [43].

It is one of the few drugs strongly recommended by the WHO [11].

4.4 Ritonavir–Lopinavir

It is a combination of drugs that aim to inhibit the protease of SARS-CoV-2 and its use was motivated by previous experiences against SARS [44]. **Figure 7** shows the chemical structure of lopinavir.

Cao et al. [44] did not find any statistically significant difference between the control and experimental group in their trial. The primary outcome they took was the decrease of two points on a severe scale or discharge. They recommend further studies to prove or discard benefits from ritonavir–lopinavir.

The WHO makes a recommendation against the use of this combination [11].

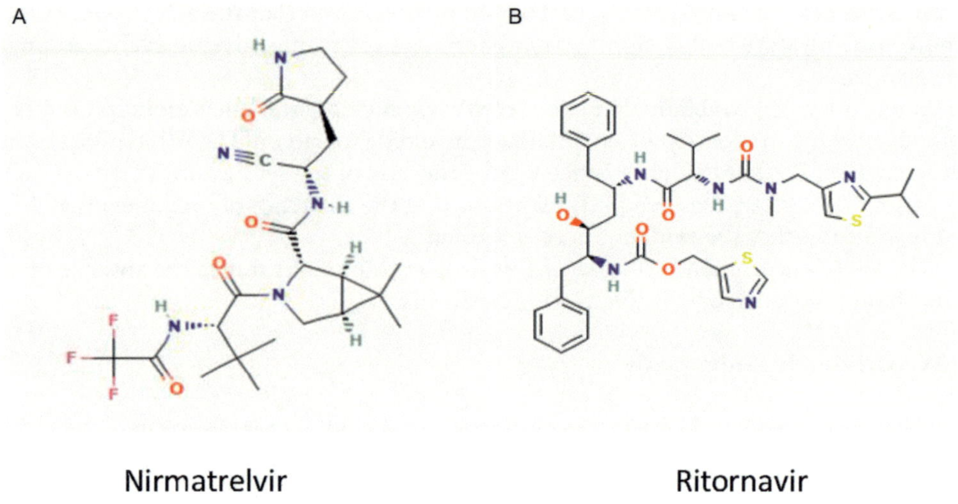

Figure 6.
Chemical structure of: (A) nirmatrelvir; and (B) ritornavir. Source: modified from PubChem. National Library of Medicine [41, 42].

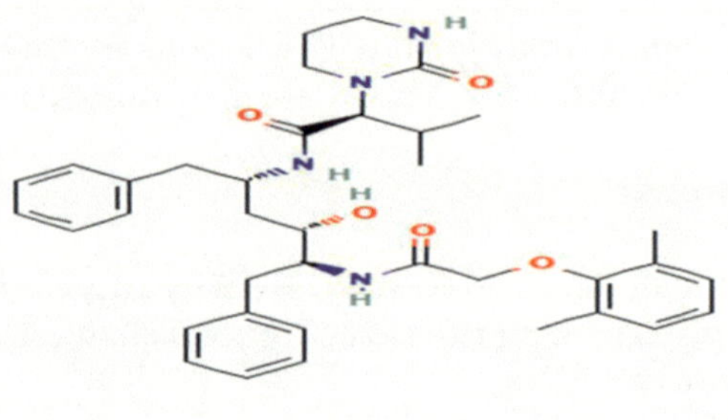

Figure 7.
Chemical structure of Lopinavir. Source: Modified from Pubchem. National Library of Medicine [45].

4.5 Remdesivir

Remdesivir is another drug that inhibits SARS-CoV-2 and was considered for its use due to previous research on its effect on SARS and MERS [46]. The chemical structure is shown in **Figure 8**.

According to Beigel et al. [46], remdesivir outperformed placebo in their clinical trial, which consisted of 1062 patients. They took discharge or hospitalization for monitoring as primary outcome. The patients in the remdesivir group reached the primary outcome approximately 5 days before the patients in the placebo group. In their trial, they administered remdesivir intravenously for three consecutive days with the following regime:

1. Day one: 200 mg

2. Day two and three: 100 mg (each day)

Wang Y et al. [48] did not find a statistically significant benefit from the use of remdesivir. Nevertheless, the samples consisted of 237 participants, and

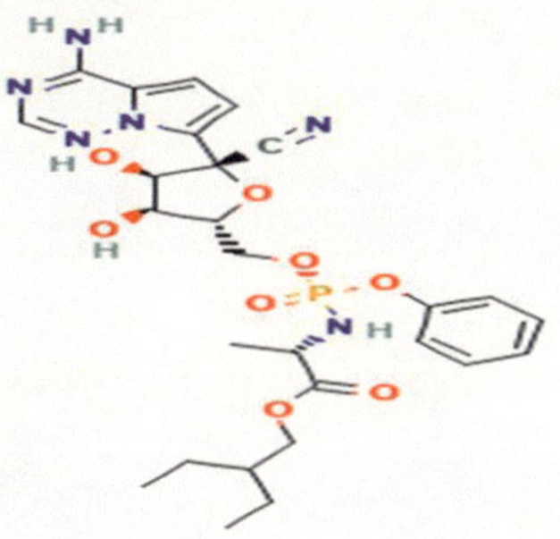

Figure 8.
Chemical structure of remdesivir. Source: Modified from Pubchem. National Library of Medicine [47].

a numerical difference among the groups was observed—supporting the use of remdesivir.

Spinner et al. [49], conducted a clinical trial comparing 5- and10-day treatment versus standard care for patients with moderate COVID-19. The differences in the primary outcome (degree on a seven-point scale) were statistically significant between the 5-day group and the standard care group. It was not observed for the differences between the 10-day group and the standard care group. Even though some results were statistically significant different, the authors are uncertain of the clinical importance.

The WHO conditionally recommends remdesivir. They suggest using it in the first 7 days after the onset of symptoms [11].

4.6 Favipiravir

Favipiravir is a drug with an active agent that halts viral replication of SARS-CoV-2 [50, 51]; its chemical structure is shown in **Figure 9**.

Manabe et al. [51] conducted a systematic review and meta-analysis on the use of favipiravir against SARS-CoV-2. They found evidence supporting the use of favipiravir to clear the virus. It was observed in various studies a viral clearance around the seventh day after the start of treatment. However, they suggest further analysis and controlled clinical trials since the evidence was heterogeneous and not straightforwardly comparable. Also, they conclude it is necessary for further research on the dose regime to have definitive conclusions.

The WHO only mentions favipiravir tangentially as a drug that might improve the outcomes by combining it with molnupiravir, observed in animal models [11].

5. On the current challenges on COVID-19 treatments

After the approval and research on treatments, there are two chief questions to address. The first question is how to distribute the drugs with equity. The other point is how they perform in the face of new SARS-CoV-2 variants.

Regarding the distribution of the treatments, the ones administered orally present clear advantages over the ones administered intravenously. Nevertheless, as pointed out by Bajaj and Stanford [53], there are important challenges to address. So far, the inequities detected are the manufacturing and pricing obstacles, and some countries buying most of the current stock [53].

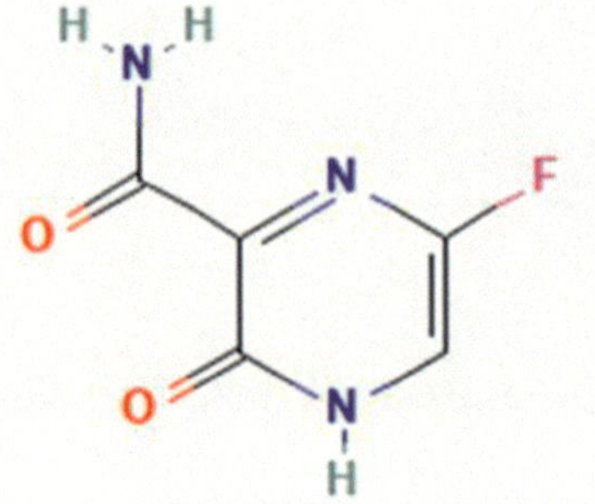

Figure 9.
Chemical structure of favipiravir. Source: Modified from Pubchem. National Library of Medicine [52].

In the face of new SARS-CoV-2, some studies have addressed the question on which therapeutics remain effective for COVID-19. According to the review made by Fernandes et al. [54], the currently approved antivirals, such as molnupiravir, ritonavir-nirmatrelvir, and remdesivir remain as effective for variants of concern as for the early versions of SARS-CoV-2. Mainly due to their mechanisms of action.

6. Conclusions

Two years ahead of the COVID-19 pandemic start, plenty of treatment options have been investigated. Only a few of them have resulted in effective and safe alternatives. The WHO [11] and the FDA [12] keep updated on the sources and status of the scientific evidence of each proposal. According to the WHO, ritonavir-nirmatrelvir outperforms other proposed therapeutics.

As SARS-CoV-2 continues mutating, an open question is whether these treatments will remain effective for these new versions. The evidence shows that they are for spike-mutated versions of the virus.

Finally, even though some drugs have been approved, availability is not even in the countries. The factors behind this include the distribution systems and logistics besides costs.

Conflict of interest

The authors declare no conflict of interest.

Author details

Nicolás Padilla-Raygoza[1*], Gilberto Flores-Vargas[1], María de Jesús Gallardo-Luna[1], Efraín Navarro-Olivos[2], Francisco Javier Magos-Vázquez[3] and Daniel Alberto Díaz-Martínez[3]

1 Department of Research and Technological Development, Directorate of Teaching and Research, Institute of Public Health from Guanajuato State, Guanajuato, Mexico

2 Directorate of Teaching and Research, Institute of Public Health from Guanajuato State, Guanajuato, Mexico

3 Directorate of Health Services, Institute of Public Health from Guanajuato State, Guanajuato, Mexico

*Address all correspondence to: npadillar@guanajuato.gob.mx

References

[1] World Health Organization. Rolling updates on coronavirus disease (COVID-19). World Health Organization. 2020. Available from: https://www.who.int/emergencies/diseases/novel-coronavirus-2019/events-as-they-happen. [Accessed: May 2, 2022]

[2] Carlos WG, De la Cruz C, Cao B, Pasnick S, Jamil S. Novel Wuhan (2019-CoV) coronavirus. American Journal of Respiratory and Critical Care Medicine. 2020;**201**(4):7-8. DOI: 10.1164/rccm.2014P7

[3] Harrison AG, Lin T, Wang P. Mechanisms of SARS-CoV-2 transmission and pathogenesis. Trends in Immunology. 2020;**41**(12):1100-1115. DOI: 10.1016/j.it.2020.10.004

[4] Sheahan TP, Sims AC, Zhou S, Graham RL, Pruijssers AJ, Agostini ML, et al. An orally bioavailable broad-spectrum antiviral inhibits SARS-CoV-2 in human airway epithelial cell cultures and multiple coronaviruses in mice. Science Translational Medicine. 2020;**12**:1-15. DOI: 10.1126/scitranslmed.abb5883

[5] Chan LYH, Yuan B, Convertino M. COVID-19 non-pharmaceutical intervention portfolio effectiveness and risk communication predominance. Scientific Reports. 2021;**11**(1):1-17. DOI: 10.1038/s41598-021-88309-1

[6] Diseases TLI. The COVID-19 infodemic. The Lancet Infectious Diseases. 2021;**20**(8):875. DOI: 10.1016/S1473-3099(20)30565-X

[7] Furlan L, Caramelli B. The regrettable story of the "Covid Kit" and the "Early Treatment of Covid-19" in Brazil. The Lancet Regional Health–Americas. 2021;**4**:100089. DOI: 10.1016/j.lana.2021.100089

[8] OMS. La OMS actualiza sus directrices terapéuticas para incluir el molnupiravir. 2022. Disponible en: https://www.who.int/es/news/item/03-03-2022-molnupiravir

[9] OMS. La OMS recomienda un tratamiento sumamente eficaz contra la COVID-19 y pide a la empresa productora amplia distribución geográfica y transparencia. 2022. Disponible en: https://www.who.int/es/news/item/22-04-2022-who-recommends-highly-successful-covid-19-therapy-and-calls-for-wide-geographical-distribution-and-transparency-from-originator

[10] Gonzalez-Canga A, Sahagun-Prieto AM, Diez-Liebana MJ, Fernandez-Martinez N, Sierra Vega M, Garcia-Vieitiz JJ. The pharmacokinetics and interactions of ivermectin in humans—A mini-review. The AAPS Journal. 2008;**10**(1):42-46. DOI: 10.1208/s12248-007-9000-9

[11] World Health Organization. Therapeutics and COVID-19: Living guideline, 22 April 2022 (No. WHO/2019-nCoV/therapeutics/2022.3). World Health Organization. Available from: https://www.who.int/publications/i/item/WHO-2019-nCoV-therapeutics-2022.3

[12] U.S. Food & Drug Administration. Coronavirus (COVID-19) | Drugs. Emergency Preparedness |Drugs. 2022. Available from: https://www.fda.gov/drugs/emergency-preparedness-drugs/coronavirus-covid-19-drugs

[13] PubChem. National Library of Medicine. Compound summary.

Ivermectin. 2022. Available from: https://pubchem.ncbi.nlm.nih.gov/compound/6321424

[14] Wagstaff KM, Rawlinson SM, Hearps AC, Jans DA. An AlphaScreen ®-based assay for high-throughput screening for specific inhibitors of nuclear import. Journal of Biomolecular Screening. 2011;**16**(2):192-200. DOI: 10.1177/1087057110390360

[15] Wagstaff KM, Sivakumaran H, Heaton SM, Harrich D, Jans DA. Ivermectin is a specific inhibitor of importin α/β-mediated nuclear import able to inhibit replication of HIV-1 and dengue virus. The Biochemical Journal. 2012;**443**(Pt. 3):851-856. DOI: 10.1042/BJ20120150

[16] Caly L, Druce JD, Catton MG, Jans DA, Wagstaff KM. The FDA-approved drug ivermectin inhibits the replication of SARS-CoV-2 in vitro. Antiviral Research. 2020;**178**:104787. DOI: 10.1016/j.antiviral.2020.104787

[17] Rajter JC, Sherman MS, Fatteh N, Vogel F, Sacks J, Rajter JJ. Use of ivermectin is associated with lower mortality in hospitalized patients with coronavirus disease 2019: The ivermectin in COVID nineteen study. Chest. 2021;**159**(1):85-92. DOI: 10.1016/j.chest.2020.10.009

[18] Siang Cob C, Merchant HA, Mustafa ZU, Shahzad HS. The association between the use of ivermectin and mortality in patients with COVID-19: A meta-analysis. Pharmacological Reports. 2021;**73**:1473-1479. DOI: 10.1007%2Fs43440-021-00245-z

[19] Bryant A, Lawrie TA, Dowswell T, Fordham EJ, Mitchell S, Hill SR, et al. Ivermectin for prevention and treatment of COVID-19 infection: A systematic review, meta-analysis, and trial sequential analysis to inform clinical guidelines. American Journal of Therapeutics. 2021;**28**(4):e434. DOI: 10.1097/MJT.0000000000001402

[20] US Food & Drug Administration. FAQ: COVID-19 and Ivermectin Intended for Animals. Available from: https://www.fda.gov/animal-veterinary/product-safety-information/faq-covid-19-and-ivermectin-intended-animals

[21] Klappenbach R, Garcia Martí S, Achon-Riviere A, Augustovski F, Alvaraz A, Bardach A, et al. Ivermectina para COVID-19. Documentos de Evaluación de Tecnologías Sanitarias. Informe de Respuesta Rápida N° 779. Argentina. 2020. Disponible: https://www.iecs.org.ar/

[22] Pan American Health Organization. World Health Organization. Ongoing living update of COVID-19 therapeutic options: Summary of evidence. PAHO. 2020. Available from: https://iris.paho.org/bitstream/handle/10665.2/52719/PAHOIMSEIHCOVID-19210001_eng.pdf?sequence=20&isAllowed=y

[23] PubChem. National Library of Medicine. Compound summary. Hydroxychloroquine. 2022. Available from: https://pubchem.ncbi.nlm.nih.gov/compound/Hydroxychloroquine

[24] RECOVERY Collaborative Group. Effect of hydroxychloroquine in hospitalized patients with Covid-19. The New England Journal of Medicine. 2020;**383**(21):2030-2040. DOI: 10.1056/NEJMoa2022926

[25] Wang M, Cao R, Zhang L, Yang X, Liu J, Xu M, et al. Remdesivir and chloroquine effectively inhibit the recently emerged novel coronavirus (2019-nCoV) in vitro. Cell Research. 2020;**30**:269-271. DOI: 10.1038/s41422-020-0282-0

[26] Schwartz IS, Boulware DR, Lee TC. Hydroxychloroquine for COVID19: The curtains close on a comedy of errors. The Lancet Regional Health–Americas. 2022;**11**:100268. Available from: https://pubmed.ncbi.nlm.nih.gov/35531052

[27] PubChem. National Library of Medicine. Compound summary. Nitazoxanide. 2022. Available from: https://pubchem.ncbi.nlm.nih.gov/compound/41684#section=2D-Structure

[28] Rosignol JF. Nitazoxanide a first-in-class broad-spectrum antiviral agent. Antiviral Research. 2014;**110**:94-103. DOI: 10.1016/j.antiviral.2014.07.014

[29] Blum VF, Cimerman S, Hunter JR, Tierno P, Lacerda A, Soeiro A, et al. Nitazoxanide superiority to placebo to treat moderate COVID-19–A Pilot prove of concept randomized double-blind clinical trial. eClinicalMedicine. 2021;**37**:100981. DOI: 10.1016/j.eclinm.2021.100981

[30] Rocco PR, Silva PL, Cruz FF, Tierno PF, Rabello E, Junior JC, et al. Nitazoxanide in patients hospitalized with COVID-19 pneumonia: A multicentre, randomized, double-blind, placebo-controlled trial. Frontiers in Medicine. 2022;**9**. DOI: 10.3389/fmed.2022.844728

[31] Oldenburg CE, Pinsky BA, Brogdon J, Chen C, Ruder K, Zhong L, et al. Effect of oral azithromycin vs placebo on COVID-19 symptoms in outpatients with SARS-CoV-2 infection: A randomized clinical trial. Journal of the American Medical Association. 2021;**326**(6):490-498. DOI: 10.1001/jama.2021.11517

[32] PubChem. National Library of Medicine. Compound summary. Azythromycin. 2022. Available from: https://pubchem.ncbi.nlm.nih.gov/compound/53477736#section=IUPAC-Name

[33] Hinks TS, Cureton L, Knight R, Wang A, Cane JL, Barber VS, et al. Azithromycin versus standard care in patients with mild-to-moderate COVID-19 (ATOMIC2): An open-label, randomised trial. The Lancet Respiratory Medicine. 2021;**9**(10):1130-1140. DOI: 10.1016/S2213-2600(21)00263-0

[34] Echeverría-Esnal D, Martin-Ontiyuelo C, Navarrete-Rouco ME, De-Antonio Cusco M, Ferrández O, Horcajada JP, et al. Azithromycin in the treatment of COVID-19: A review. Expert Review of Anti-Infective Therapy. 2021;**19**(2):147-163. DOI: 10.1080/14787210.2020.1813024

[35] Singh AK, Singh A, Singh R, Misra A. Molnupiravir in COVID-19: A systematic review of literature. Diabetes and Metabolic Syndrome: Clinical Research and Reviews. 2021;**15**(6):102329. DOI: 10.1016/j.dsx.2021.102329

[36] PubChem. National Library of Medicine. Compound summary. Molnupiravir. 2022. Available from: https://pubchem.ncbi.nlm.nih.gov/compound/145996610#section=2D-Structure

[37] Jayk Bernal A, Gomes da Silva MM, Musungaie DB, Kovalchuk E, Gonzalez A, Delos Reyes V, et al. Molnupiravir for oral treatment of Covid-19 in nonhospitalized patients. The New England Journal of Medicine. 2022;**386**(6):509-520. DOI: 10.1056/NEJMoa2116044

[38] Extance A. Covid-19: What is the evidence for the antiviral molnupiravir? BMJ. 2022;**377**:o926. DOI: 10.1136/bmj.o926

[39] Abani O, Abbas A, Abbas F, Abbas M, Abbasi S, Abbass H, et al. Casirivimab and imdevimab in patients admitted to hospital with COVID-19 (RECOVERY): A randomised, controlled, open-label, platform trial. The Lancet. 2022;**399**(10325):665-676. DOI: 10.1016/S0140-6736(22)00163-5

[40] Hammond J, Leister-Tebbe H, Gardner A, Abreu P, Bao W, Wisemandle W, et al. Oral nirmatrelvir for high-risk, nonhospitalized adults with COVID-19. The New England Journal of Medicine. 2022;**386**(15):1397-1408. DOI: 10.1056/NEJMoa2118542

[41] PubChem. National Library of Medicine. Compound summary. Nirmatrelvir. 2022. Available from: https://pubchem.ncbi.nlm.nih.gov/compound/155903259

[42] PubChem. National Library of Medicine. Compound summary. Ritonavir. 2022. Available from: https://pubchem.ncbi.nlm.nih.gov/compound/392622#section=2D-Structure

[43] Lamb YN. Nirmatrelvir plus Ritonavir: First approval. Drugs. 2022;**82**(5):585-591. DOI: 10.1007/s40265-022-01692-5

[44] Cao B, Wang Y, Wen D, Liu W, Wang J, Fan G, et al. A trial of lopinavir–ritonavir in adults hospitalized with severe Covid-19. The New England Journal of Medicine. 2020;**382**:1787-1799. DOI: 10.1056/NEJMoa2001282

[45] PubChem. National Library of Medicine. Compound summary. Lopinavir. 2022. Available from: https://pubchem.ncbi.nlm.nih.gov/compound/92727#section=2D-Structure

[46] Beigel JH, Tomashek KM, Dodd LE, Metha AK, Zingman BS, Kalil AC, et al. Remdesivir for the treatment of Covid-19—final report. The New England Journal of Medicine. 2020;**383**(19):1813-1826. DOI: 10.1056/NEJMoa2007764

[47] PubChem. National Library of Medicine. Compound summary. Remdesivir. 2022. Available from: https://pubchem.ncbi.nlm.nih.gov/compound/121304016#section=2D-Structure

[48] Wang Y, Zhang D, Du G, Du R, Zhao J, Jin Y, et al. Remdesivir in adults with severe COVID-19: A randomised, double-blind, placebo-controlled, multicentre trial. The Lancet. 2020;**395**(10236):1569-1578. DOI: 10.1016/S0140-6736(20)31022-9

[49] Spinner CD, Gottlieb RL, Criner GJ, López JRA, Cattelan AM, Viladomiu AS, et al. Effect of remdesivir vs standard care on clinical status at 11 days in patients with moderate COVID-19: A randomized clinical trial. Journal of the American Medical Association. 2020;**324**(11):1048-1057. DOI: 10.1001/jama.2020.16349

[50] Furuta Y, Komeno T, Nakamura T. Favipiravir (T-705), a broad spectrum inhibitor of viral RNA polymerase. Proceedings of the Japan Academy, Series B. 2017;**93**(7):449-463. DOI: 10.2183%2Fpjab.93.027

[51] Manabe T, Kambayashi D, Akatsu H, Kudo K. Favipiravir for the treatment of patients with COVID-19: A systematic review and meta-analysis. BMC Infectious Diseases. 2021;**21**(1):1-13. DOI: 10.1186/s12879-021-06164-x

[52] PubChem. National Library of Medicine. Compound summary. Favipiravir. 2022. Available from: https://pubchem.ncbi.nlm.nih.gov/compound/492405#section=2D-Structure

[53] Bajaj SS, Stanford FC. COVID-19: LMICs need antivirals as well as vaccines. Nature. 2022;**602**(7895):33. DOI: 10.1038/d41586-022-00220-5

[54] Fernandes Q, Philipose Inchakalody V, Merhi M, Mestiri S, Taib N, Abo El-Ella DM, et al. Emerging COVID-19 variants and their impact on SARS-CoV-2 diagnosis, therapeutics and vaccines. Annals of Medicine. 2022;**54**(1):524-540. DOI: 10.1080/07853890.2022.2031274

Chapter 6

Inclusive Review on Existing Treatment and Management Modalities for COVID-19

Jalpa Suthar and Jhanvi Patel

Abstract

COVID 19 is widely regarded as one of the worst pandemics of the twenty-first century. The World Health Organization (WHO) named the viral infection caused by the new coronavirus (COVID-19), which was first reported in December 2019, as severe acute respiratory syndrome-Coronavirus-2 (SARS-CoV2), and it became a cause of death for many all over the world. As a result, a unique inquiry and clinical trial to find a solution for this catastrophic pandemic disease is under way. To manage and eradicate the disease, effective vaccinations and antiviral therapies are urgently needed. There were no treatments or vaccines available for this fatal virus at first, but several medications that are used to treat other diseases are now being used to treat Covid19. Remdesivir has been licenced for therapy since it has shown to shorten hospital stays. Corticosteroids reduced mortality in patients requiring oxygen supplementation or mechanical ventilation. The purpose of this review is to make readers aware of the possible efficacy and availability treatment for this viral infection.

Keywords: COVID-19, severe acute respiratory syndrome, corticosteroids, remdesivir, first wave, second wave

1. Introduction

Covid-19 which is also known as novel coronavirus pneumonia firstly encountered in Wuhan, China in December 2019. The WHO Emergency committee declared a global health emergency on 30 January 2020 based on the growing case rates of covid-19 at Chinese and international locations [1]. This virus spread was so rapid that after 2 weeks from the first case diagnosed, 1000 patients were tested positive and the number of positive cases reached over 30,000 and 2500 deaths by 18, March 2020 [2].

The rate at which transmission of nCoV19 among the human is increasing than SARS CoV1 and MERS CoV, one of the group of international committee on taxonomy of virus (ICTV) named as coronaviridae study group (CSG) renamed as SARS CoV2, while WHO named as Coronavirus disease 2019 (COVID-19) [3]. Structurally SARS CoV2 contains single strand RNA [4] of which two third part of RNA is located in open reading frame (ORF) which include polyproteins and non-structural protein for viral cycle [3]. There are other structural protein which are encoded by ORF's like spike glycoprotein (S), enveloped protein (E), matrix protein (M) and nucleocapsid protein (N). S protein of virus attached to host cell's receptor is present on the angiotensin converting enzyme 2 (ACE2) [5] from which SARS CoV2 passes through the mucous membrane of respiratory tract from which it enter to lungs then to systemic circulation through which it could target organ such as heart, brain, renal, lungs, GIT [3]. Then after entering into the cell, it gets replicated using protein such as chymotrypsin(proteases) and RNA polymerase.

The number of COVID-19 cases in second wave was much higher than the first wave of COVID-19. There were several factors responsible for the same. There are some clear distinctions between the first and second waves which are shown in **Table 1**. Paediatric and younger people, as well as older people, got infected in the second wave. COVID 2nd wave symptoms were extremely varied [6].

From an Indian standpoint, things moved slowly initially, with the first cases showing in February 2020. The lockdown had its drawbacks, in that it controlled the disease to a certain level in the hopes of a few treatments fighting against the virus. Hydroxychloroquine, azithromycin, favipiravir, an antiviral, and ivermectin, an anthelminthic, were being used during the start of the pandemic in India [7].

The majority of COVID-19 patients had mild-to-moderate symptoms and were treated by qualified clinicians outside of the hospital. In India, a typical COVID-19 prescription contains azithromycin, doxycycline, ivermectin, hydroxychloroquine, vitamin C, vitamin D, zinc, acetylcysteine, and budesonide inhalation or dexamethasone [8].

Despite not being indicated for COVID-19 by any major standards, the antiviral favipiravir became India's best-selling medicine in April 2021. Despite the advice of most international expert panels, anticoagulants like rivaroxaban were prescribed in outpatient settings, even for patients with no elevated thrombotic risk. Antibiotics with a broad spectrum of action are introduced under the pretence of treating secondary infections [8].

There has never been a poly-prescription of the mentioned medications previously. It's unclear how these pharmaceuticals interact with one another (or with medications administered for pre-existing problems). It becomes difficult to tell whether a new symptom is caused by COVID-19 progression, an adverse drug reaction, or a new consequence [8].

Due to structural similarities of SARS CoV2 to HIV, Hepatitis B, C the drugs used for the treatment of Hepatitis C virus [4] i.e. remdesivir is also used in SARS CoV2 as antiviral agents. Hence nucleoside analogues HIV proteases inhibitors (also RNA Polymerase) may be useful in COVID 19. On the other hand the second antiviral drug used in COVID treatment is FAVIPIRAVIR which is a purine based analogue [9] and RNA dependent RNA polymerase (RdRp) inhibitors which will inhibit RdRp for transcription and replication of viral genomes [3]. An another purine nucleoside analogue ribavirin, inhibits the activity of enzyme IMPDH [9] (Inosine-5-monophosphate dehydrogenase) which leads to the suppression of the cellular DNA and mRNA which lead to suppression of protein synthesis, due to deceased level of the intracellular guanosine triphosphate pool.

Apart from this other two methods were also used for hindering the replication which included immune modulation where convalescent plasma therapy was used [10] and viral entry inhibition which was achieved by drug hydroxychloroquine (HCQ) [9]. Hydroxychloroquine and chloroquine which are anti-malarial agents with anti-inflammatory activities, can produce immune modulatory effect too, therefore

	First wave	**Second wave**
Causative organism	SARS-Cov-2 virus	Various mutants of SARS-Cov-2 virus
Knowledge about the disease	Less	More knowledge
Symptomatology	Mostly related to respiratory system	New symptoms like Gastrointestinal etc.
Presentation	More severe	Less intense
Shortness of breath	Fewer cases with breathlessness	Much more cases with breathlessness
Age profile of the patients	Elder patients widely affected	Effect seen more in younger patients
Comorbidities	Patients with comorbidities affected more	Less
Drug availability	Acute shortage and black marketing	Available in the hospitals and pharmacies
Health care workers	They were lesser trained, not vaccinated and afraid of acquiring infection	• More trained increased • Lesser fear to acquire infection • Mostly vaccinated
Bed capacity	Limited	Enhanced
Ventilator beds	Less than 25,000	Increased to more than 50,000
Laboratory testing	Only one laboratory in January 2020	More laboratories in Private and Government center
PPE	Scarcity	Plenty 1 million PPE produced
Vaccine	Not available	Approved vaccines available
Treatment affordability	• Increased test price • Increased treatment cost and PPE	• Markedly reduced test price • Reduced treatment cost and PPE
Oxygen requirement to the patient	Less	More
Requirement of mechanical ventilation	Less	More
Disease Spread	Slower	Much faster
Plasma Therapy	Limited	Much more
Death rate	Higher	Lower
Positivity rate	Lower	Much higher

Table 1.
Differences between the first and the second wave of COVID-19 in India.

a useful option for COVID 19 management. HCQ is known to demonstrate high potency inhibition of SARS CoV 2 virus in invitro studies. Besides this, corticosteroids also showed a tendency to reduce or prevent the systemic inflammation seen in COVID 19 patients [9]. Additionally many other drugs have also been selected for managing COVID 19 infection like Azithromycin (as antibiotics) lopinavir-ritonavir, interferon (antiviral drugs) multivitamins (vitamin D, vitamin C, and zinc) [3, 4, 9]. The supportive treatments included non-pharmacological approaches.

The C reactive protein and serum albumin have shown independent prognostic marker along with the age, maximum body temperature, smoking status and respiratory failure [11]. The immune response of the patients is weakened by inadequate nutrition. This shows that the nutritional derangements should be systematically managed in patients suffering from coronavirus. Besides giving the medicines or drugs when the patient's body is not responding to medications the other therapy used was convalescent plasma therapy where the plasma from recovered patients was ejected out and given to the infected one [12]. Vaccination helped to improve the immune system of individuals [13].

The review emphasis on the comprehensive overview on various treatment modalities available for the management of Covid-19.

2. Drug treatment options available for Covid-19 treatment and management

2.1 Drug treatment for Mild to moderate Covid-19 infection

2.1.1 Molnupiravir

Molnupiravir is an orally accessible prodrug of the nucleoside analogue -D-N4-hydroxycytidine and is a broad-spectrum antiviral (NHC). In replicating coronaviruses, molnupiravir or NHC can promote G to A and C to U transition mutations [14].

Mechanism of action: NHC circulates systemically after molnupiravir dosing and is phosphorylated intracellularly to NHC triphosphate. Viral RNA polymerase incorporates NHC triphosphate into viral RNA, which then misdirects viral polymerase to incorporate either guanosine or adenosine during viral replication. As a result, detrimental mistakes accumulate throughout the viral genome, rendering the virus non-infectious and unable to replicate [15].

Adverse effects: Diarrhea, Dizziness and Nausea [16].

Other indications: NA.

2.1.2 Azithromycin

Azithromycin is a broad-spectrum macrolide antibiotic with a protracted half-existence and tremendous tissue penetration. It is mostly used for the remedy of respiration, enteric and genitourinary infections and can be utilized in desire to different macrolides for a few sexually transmitted and enteric infections. Azithromycin has extra immunomodulatory consequences and has been utilized in continual respiration inflammatory illnesses for this purpose [17].

Mechanism of action: Azithromycin has antiviral action against SARS-CoV-2 and may act at various stages of the viral cycle. Its immunomodulatory features include the capacity to reduce cytokine production, maintain epithelial cell integrity, and prevent fibrosis in the lungs [18].

Adverse effects: QTc prolongation has been linked to torsade's de pointes and polymorphic ventricular tachycardia, rarely hepatotoxicity [18].

Other indications: Community-acquired pneumonia, in relation to its activity against Streptococcus pneumoniae, Hemophilus influenzae, and Moraxella catarrhalis. Treatment of other upper respiratory diseases, like acute otitis media and acute reoccurrence of chronic obstructive pulmonary disease [19].

2.1.3 Favipiravir

Favipiravir is an oral medication that was authorized in Japan in 2014 for new and re-emerging pandemic influenza. Favipiravir (prodrug) is a purine base analogue that undergoes intracellular phosphoribosylation to become active favipiravir ribofuranosyl-5B triphosphate (favipiravir-RTP).

Mechanism of action: Favipiravir is integrated into the nascent viral RNA via the error-prone viral RdRp, resulting in viral mutagenesis and chain termination. The presence of RdRp in many types of RNA viruses allows favipiravir to have a broader spectrum of antiviral activity. Favipiravir-RTP acts as a mutagen after RNA viral inclusion, allowing it to avoid coronavirus repair machinery. Overall, favipiravir-RTP has a beneficial effect on SARS-CoV-2 by inducing a cytopathic effect, which reduces the number of viral RNA and infectious particles, as well as increasing the frequency of mutation [20].

Adverse effects: Abnormal liver function tests, psychiatric symptom reactions, digestive tract reactions and raised serum uric acid [3].

Other indications: RNA viruses such as resistant influenzas virus, arenaviruses, Bunyaviruses, floviruses, Rift Valley Fever, Yellow Fever, West Nile, Western equine encephalitis, foot-and-mouth disease virus, norovirus and avian influenza [3].

2.1.4 JAK-STAT inhibitors

As cytokines are clearly important in the fight against viral infections, the hyperinflammatory conditions caused by the SARS-CoV-2 infection due to the cytokine storm.

Mechanism of action: STAT proteins with SH2 domains are inactive and restricted to the cytoplasm in unstimulated cells. STAT proteins use SH2 domains to bind to the phospho-tyrosine that includes receptor sequences after cytokine receptor stimulation. Furthermore, JAK-induced phosphorylation of STAT proteins at cytokine type receptors results in STAT protein dimerization. STATs can translocate inside the nucleus and trigger apoptosis, immunological modulation, cell cycle differentiation, and gene transcription due to their dimerization.

Adverse effects: Ruxolitinib: Purpuric lesions on the skin of limbs and erythrodermic rashes in 2 SARS-CoV-2 patients.

Long term use of Baricitinib: Serious infections and thromboembolic events in patients.

Tofacitinib: Abdominal pain, acne vulgaris, anemia, angioedema, diarrhea, dehydration, dyspepsia, headache, hepatotoxicity, hyperlipidemia, hepatitis, lymphoma, lymphopenia, nausea, neutropenia, pulmonary embolism, rashes, vomiting, blood clots, GI perforations [21].

Other indications: Rheumatoid arthritis, Psoriatic arthritis, Ulcerative Colitis, Chron's disease, Alopecia areata, Vitiligo, Psoriasis, Atopic dermatitis [22].

2.2 Drug treatment for severe Covid-19 infection

2.2.1 Remdesivir

Remdesivir (RDV), also known as GS-5734, is a monophosphoramidate prodrug and adenosine nucleoside analogue that is converted to GS-441524, the active form [3].

Mechanism of action: Remdesivir inhibits viral RNA-dependent RNA polymerase (RdRp), which is involved in viral genome replication. When remdesivir is metabolized by the host cells into its pharmacologic active analogue, adenosine triphosphate (GS-443902), it competes with ATP for integration by the RdRp complex into the nascent RNA strand, resulting in the cessation of RNA synthesis and reducing viral replication [23].

Adverse effects: Hypotension, arrhythmias, and cardiac arrest, Dyspnea, Acute respiratory failure, acute respiratory distress, pneumothorax, pulmonary embolism, Anemia, lymphopenia, Hyperglycemia, Pneumonia, septic shock, Elevated lipase, nausea, vomiting, diarrhea, constipation, poor appetite, gastroparesis, and lower GI bleeding, Acute kidney injury or worsening of underlying chronic kidney disease, hypernatremia, hypokalemia, Headache, lightheadedness, Rash, contact dermatitis, pruritus, Delirium, Pyrexia, insomnia, multi-organ dysfunction and DVT.

Other indication: Ebola Virus [24].

2.2.2 Dexamethasone

Dexamethasone is a corticosteroid with anti-inflammatory and immunosuppressive properties that is used to treat a variety of illnesses [25].

Mechanism of action: It works by blockade of inflammation pathways, vasodilation and immune cell migration [26].

Adverse effects: Hyperglycemia, secondary infections, psychiatric effects, avascular necrosis [25].

Other indications: Allergic states, GIT disorders, Hematologic disorder, Renal disorders [25].

2.2.3 Selinexor

Selinexor, a selective inhibitor of nuclear localization compound that structures exportin 1 (XPO1) and compels nuclear concentration and initiation of oncogenic proteins, inhibits transcription factor nf B, and reduces oncoprotein messenger RNA translation, could be a new treatment option for myeloma that has resisted current treatments [27].

Mechanism of action: The severe pulmonary inflammation associated with COVID-19, as well as high levels of cytokines such as IL6, IL1, IFNg, and others, is one of the most essential features of the virus. Selinexor has shown substantial anti-inflammatory effect by inhibiting Nuclear Factor kB (NF-kB), resulting in decreases in all of these cytokines and is helpful especially for COVID-19 patients who are hospitalized [28].

Adverse effects: Blurred vision, Cataract was reported as the most widespread side effect [29]. Nausea, vomiting, diarrhea, constipation, weight loss. Loss of appetite. Extreme tiredness. Difficulty falling asleep or staying asleep. Headache. taste changes. Easy bleeding or bruising, fatigue, pale skin, or shortness of breath, fever, cough, chills, or other signs of infection, seeing things or hearing voices that do not exist, confusion, double vision and increased sensitivity to light and glare [30].

Other indications: Selinexor is indicated for the remedy of relapsed or refractory a couple of myelomas in aggregate with dexamethasone. Patients need to have acquired as a minimum four previous treatments and feature sickness that's refractory to least proteasome inhibitors, as a minimum immunomodulatory agent, and an anti-CD38 monoclonal antibody [31].

2.2.4 Nitric oxide

In the cardiovascular and immune systems, nitric oxide plays a significant pathophysiological role. NO works as a selective pulmonary vasodilator to promote oxygenation and lessen pulmonary vascular resistance [32].

Mechanism of action: NO has the ability to act as a vasodilator and immunological regulator. As a vasodilator, it works as a selective pulmonary vasodilator to improve oxygenation and reduce pulmonary vascular resistance, as a bronchial/airway dilator to promote oxygen inhalation, as a vascular anticoagulant to prevent blood clotting and excessive platelet activation [33].

Adverse effects: Blurred vision, dizziness, faintness, or light-headedness. Sweating, Unusual exhaustion or weakness. Incidence not known: bluish lips or skin, Chest discomfort, Difficult or labored breathing, Dizziness, Tightness in the chest, Trouble breathing [33]. Clinical adverse effects of iNO include the following: Worsening heart failure, Hypotension, Pulmonary vasospasm, Methemoglobinemia [34, 35].

Other indications: Pulmonary Hypertension in Infants, Chronic Lung Disease in the Infant [34]. Improve oxygenation and reduce the risk of extracorporeal membrane oxygenation in term and near-term infants with hypoxic respiratory failure and clinical and/or echocardiographic signs of pulmonary hypertension [35].

2.2.5 Paxlovid

Ritonavir-Boosted Nirmatrelvir. Nirmatrelvir is an orally absorbed protease inhibitor that inhibits MPRO, a viral protease that cleaves the two viral polyproteins required for viral replication. It has shown antiviral activity against all known coronaviruses that infect people [36].

Mechanism of action: Paxlovid is made up of two drugs: nirmatrelvir, which stops the virus from replicating by inhibiting a SARS-CoV-2 protein, and ritonavir, which slows down the breakdown of nirmatrelvir and allows it to stay in the body for longer at higher concentrations [37].

Adverse effects: Diarrhea, Altered or impaired sense of taste, Muscle aches, Increased blood pressure [38].

2.3 Supportive treatments for Covid-19 infection

2.3.1 Paracetamol

Paracetamol, often known as acetaminophen, is a pain reliever and fever reducer commonly used for mild to moderate pain and discomfort. This medicine has been prescribed to alleviate the symptoms of COVID-19 infection, which include fever, body aches, and headaches. Patients with these symptoms may find relief with paracetamol, but it is not a treatment for COVID-19 [39].

Adverse effects: Itchy, red, swollen, blistered, or peeling skin, wheezing, chest or throat tightness, difficulty breathing or speaking, swelling of the mouth, face, lips, tongue, or throat [40].

2.3.2 Vitamin D

It has the ability to function autocrinally in a local immunologic environment. Vitamin D has the ability to influence both innate and adaptive immune responses. Vitamin D deficiency has been linked to increased autoimmunity and susceptibility to infection. As immune cells in autoimmune diseases are responsive to the ameliorative effects of vitamin D, the beneficial effects of supplementing vitamin D-deficient individuals with autoimmune disease may extend beyond the effects on bone and calcium homeostasis [41].

Mechanism of action: Vitamin D receptors are found on B cells, T cells, and antigen-presenting cells, among other immune cells. Because these cells may generate the active vitamin D metabolite, vitamin D has the potential to manipulate innate and adaptive immune responses [42].

Adverse effects: Some side effects of taking too much vitamin D include weakness, dry mouth, nausea, vomiting, and others. Taking vitamin D for long periods of time in doses higher than 4000 IU (100 mcg) daily is possibly unsafe and may cause very high levels of calcium in the blood [43].

Other indications: Osteoporosis, Hypoparathyroidism, Vitamin D resistant Rickets, Familial Hypophosphatemia [44].

2.3.3 Vitamin C

Vitamin C levels in serum and leukocytes are depleted during the acute stage of infection owing to increased metabolic demands. Vitamin C supplementation at a high dose aid in the normalization of serum and leukocyte vitamin C levels. Vitamin C has a number of pharmacological properties, including antiviral, anti-oxidant, anti-inflammatory, and immunomodulatory activities, making it a promising treatment choice for COVID-19 [45].

Mechanism of action: Vitamin C, also known as ascorbic acid, is a water-soluble nutrient that is vital for human health. Immune responses rely heavily on ascorbic acid. As an antioxidant, vitamin C plays a vital homeostatic role. It has been shown to have direct virucidal activity as well as increase interferon production. Both the innate and adaptive immune systems have effector mechanisms. Vitamin C inhibits NF-B activation, which reduces reactive oxidative species (ROS) and inflammation. While SARS-CoV-2 suppresses the expression of type-1 interferons (the host's main antiviral defense), ascorbic acid increases the expression of these important host defense proteins [46].

Adverse effects: Nausea, vomiting and diarrhea, Heartburn, Stomach cramps or bloating, Fatigue and sleepiness, or sometimes insomnia, Headache, Skin flushing. Vitamin C supplements taken orally, especially in large doses, might produce kidney stones. The use of oral vitamin C supplements in excess of 2000 milligrams per day for an extended period of time raises the risk of serious side effects [47].

Other indication: Assisting in the protection and maintenance of cells. Maintaining healthy skin, blood vessels, bones and cartilage. Assisting in the healing of wounds [48].

2.3.4 Zinc

Zinc is a trace mineral, which means it is only needed in minute amounts by the body, yet it is required for almost 100 enzymes to carry out critical chemical reactions. It plays an important role in the formation of DNA, cell development, protein synthesis, tissue repair, and immune system support [49].

Mechanism of action: Zn supplementation has the ability to increase innate and humoral antiviral immunity, as well as restore reduced immune cell activity or improve normal immune cell function, especially in immunocompromised or elderly patients. When used with normal antiviral therapy, Zn has been shown to have a synergistic effect in patients with hepatitis C, HIV, and SARS-CoV-1. Physical processes such as virus adhesion, infection, and uncoating are primarily responsible for Zn's effectiveness against a variety of viral species. Zn may also protect or stabilize the cell membrane, which may help to prevent the virus from entering the cell [50].

Adverse effects: Indigestion, Diarrhea, Headache, Nausea, Vomiting [51].

Other indications: Zinc can be used to treat zinc deficiency, diarrhea, and Wilson disease. Acne, diabetes, anorexia, burns, and a variety of other conditions are all treated with zinc. Several scientific evidence supports its usage in the treatment of some of these conditions [52].

Additionally, supplemental oxygen therapy is provided to patients with Severe Covid and respiratory distress, hypoxemia, or shock. Oxygen therapy at 5 L/min and titrate flow rates to reach target SpO2 ≥ 90% in non-pregnant adults and SpO2 ≥ 92–96% in pregnant patients. NIV/HFNC (Helmet or face mask interface depending on availability) should be used in patients with increasing oxygen requirement, if work of breathing is increasing.

Intubation should be prioritized in patients with high work of breathing /if NIV is not tolerated., presence of hemodynamic instability, altered mental status or multi-organ failure. Ventilatory management carried out according to protocol [53].

3. Standard treatment according to MoHFW for different severities of COVID-19 infection

MoHFW (Ministry of Health and Family Welfare) is a government ministry in India that is responsible for health policy [53]. It is also in charge of all government-sponsored family planning programmes in India. As a member of the Council of Ministers, the Minister of Health and Family Welfare has cabinet rank.

The standard treatment given by MoHFW for different severities is given below.

Drug treatment for patients with mild cases:

i. Tab Paracetamol for fever and if fever is not controlled with a maximum dose of Tab. Paracetamol 650 mg QDS, then consult a doctor and they may prescribe drugs like non-steroidal anti-inflammatory drug like for example Tab.Naproxen 250 mg twice a day.

ii. Tab Ivermectin (200 mcg/kg OD) for 3–5 days (avoid in pregnant and lactating women)

iii. Tab Hydroxychloroquine (400 mg BD for 1 day, followed by 400 mg daily for next 4 days, unless contraindicated)

iv. Inhalational Budesonide (given via inhalers with spacer at a dose of 800 mcg BD for 5–7 days) only to be given if symptoms (fever and/or cough) are persistent beyond 5 days of disease onset.

v. Systemic oral steroids not required in mild severity. If symptoms are persistent beyond 7 days (persistent fever, worsening cough etc.) consult the doctor for treatment with low dose oral steroids.

vi. Continue the medications for other co-morbidities.

Drug Treatment for patients with moderate cases:

i. Antipyretic (Paracetamol) for fever and pain,

ii. Anti- tussives for cough

iii. Adequate hydration should be ensured

iv. Oxygen Support: Target SpO2: 92–96% (88–92% with COPD patients). The device chosen for administering oxygen depends on the severity of hypoxia and work of breathing.

v. Anticoagulants: Prophylactic dose of Un-Fractionated Heparin (UFH) or Low Molecular Weight Heparin (LMWH) (e.g., enoxaparin 0.5 mg/Kg body wt per day SC). Consider UFH in ESRD.

vi. Anti-inflammatory or immunomodulatory therapy: IV Methylprednisolone 0.5–1 mg/kg OR IV Dexamethasone 0.1–0.2 mg/kg for a duration of 5–10 days. Switch to oral therapy if the patient's health is improving.

vii. Antibiotics should be prescribed only when clinical suspicion of bacterial infection. Those who develop infection, consider empiric antibiotic therapy as per local antibiogram.

viii. Continue the medications for other co-morbidities.

Drug treatment for patients with severe cases:

i. Symptomatic treatment with paracetamol,

ii. Antitussives for cough

iii. When no evidence of shock use of conservative fluid management in patients to maintain euvolemia.

iv. Respiratory support according to the requirement.

v. Anti-inflammatory or immunomodulatory therapy: IV Methylprednisolone 1–2 mg/kg IV in two divided doses (or 0.2–0.4 mg/kg of dexamethasone) usually for 5–10 days.

vi. Anticoagulants: Prophylactic dose of Un-Fractionated Heparin (UFH) or Low Molecular Weight Heparin (LMWH) (e.g., enoxaparin 0.5 mg/Kg body wt per day SC). Consider UFH in ESRD.

To conclude, these are the drugs that are used in India for the treatment of mild, moderate and severe covid infection. For mild-moderate infection, Molnupiravir, Azithromycin, JAK-STAT Inhibitors and Favipiravir. For severe covid infections, drugs like Remdesivir, Paxlovid, Nitric Oxide, Selinexor and Dexamethasone. Common treatment includes Nutritional and Vitamin Supplements, Paracetamol and Zinc. Additionally,Nitazoxanide, Niclosamide, Rintatolimod, Bencentinib, Plitidepsin, VIR-2703, Emetine hydrochloride, AT-527, Trabedersen, Stannous protoporphyrin, Antroquinonol, Apilimod dimesylate, Brilacidin, Infliximab, Abatacept, Cenicriviroc, Interleukin-1 inhibitors, Interleukin-7 inhibitors are drugs under trial for the treatment for COVID 19 infection. As per the latest data from WHO, the total confirmed cases since the pandemic started till May end 2022 are 43,147,530 and the total deaths accounts to 524,539 [54].

Author details

Jalpa Suthar* and Jhanvi Patel
Department of Pharmacology, Ramanbhai Patel College of Pharmacy, Charotar University of Science and Technology (CHARUSAT), Changa, India

*Address all correspondence to: jalpasuthar.ph@charusat.ac.in

References

[1] Velavan TP, Meyer CG. The COVID-19 epidemic. Tropical Medicine & International Health. 2020;**25**(3):278

[2] Spinelli A, Pellino G. COVID-19 pandemic: Perspectives on an unfolding crisis. Journal of British Surgery. 2020;**107**(7):785-787

[3] Sahebnasagh A, Avan R, Saghafi F, Mojtahedzadeh M, Sadremomtaz A, Arasteh O, et al. Pharmacological treatments of COVID-19. Pharmacological Reports. 2020;**72**(6):1

[4] Raghunathan V, Dhaliwal M. Pharmacological management of COVID-19. Journal of Pediatric Critical Care. 2020;**7**(7):42

[5] Dias PGI, RMUSK R. Transmission, stability, symptoms, diagnosis and management of COVID 19. Asian Journal of Research in Infectious Diseases. 2020;**4**:39-47

[6] Jain VK, Iyengar KP, Vaishya R. Differences between First wave and Second wave of COVID-19 in India. Diabetes & Metabolic Syndrome. 2021;**15**(3):1047

[7] Allam M, Cai S, Ganesh S, Venkatesan M, Doodhwala S, Song Z, et al. COVID-19 diagnostics, tools, and prevention. Diagnostics. 2020;**10**(6). Available from: /pmc/articles/PMC7344926/

[8] Bhaumik S, John O, Jha V. Low-value medical care in the pandemic-is this what the doctor ordered? The Lancet Global Health. 2021;**9**(9):e1203-e1204

[9] Drożdżal S, Rosik J, Lechowicz K, Machaj F, Kotfis K, Ghavami S, et al. FDA approved drugs with pharmacotherapeutic potential for SARS-CoV-2 (COVID-19) therapy. Drug Resistance Updates: Reviews and Commentaries in Antimicrobial and Anticancer Chemotherapy. 2020;**53**

[10] G P. Treatment modalities for coronavirus disease 2019 (COVID-19). Journal of Medical and Scientific Research. 2020;**8**(S1):106-111

[11] Mahmood Z, Alrefai H, Hetta HF, Kader HA, Munawar N, Rahman SA, et al. Investigating virological, immunological, and pathological avenues to identify potential targets for developing COVID-19 treatment and prevention strategies. Vaccines. 2020;**8**(3):443

[12] Habas K, Nganwuchu C, Shahzad F, Gopalan R, Haque M, Rahman S, et al. Resolution of coronavirus disease 2019 (COVID-19). 2020;**18**(12):1201-1211. DOI: 101080/14787210202017974\87

[13] Caccialanza R, Laviano A, Lobascio F, Montagna E, Bruno R, Ludovisi S, et al. Early nutritional supplementation in non-critically ill patients hospitalized for the 2019 novel coronavirus disease (COVID-19): Rationale and feasibility of a shared pragmatic protocol. Nutrition (Burbank, Los Angeles County, Calif). 2020:74

[14] Gordon CJ, Tchesnokov EP, Schinazi RF, Götte M. Molnupiravir promotes SARS-CoV-2 mutagenesis via the RNA template. The Journal of Biological Chemistry. 2021;**297**(1)

[15] Jayk Bernal A, Gomes da Silva MM, Musungaie DB, Kovalchuk E, Gonzalez A, Delos Reyes V, et al. Molnupiravir for oral treatment of Covid-19 in nonhospitalized patients. New England Journal of Medicine. 2022;**386**(6):509-520

[16] 9 Things You Need To Know About Molnupiravir, a New COVID-19 Pill > News > Yale Medicine. Available from: https://www.yalemedicine.org/news/9-things-to-know-about-covid-pill

[17] McMullan BJ, Mostaghim M. Prescribing azithromycin. Australian Prescriber. 2015;**38**(3):87

[18] Echeverría-Esnal D, Martin-Ontiyuelo C, Navarrete-Rouco ME, De-Antonio Cuscó M, Ferrández O, Horcajada JP, et al. Azithromycin in the treatment of COVID-19: A review. Expert Review of Anti-Infective Therapy. 2021;**19**(2):147-163

[19] Azithromycin (Oral Route)—Mayo Clinic

[20] Joshi S, Parkar J, Ansari A, Vora A, Talwar D, Tiwaskar M, et al. Role of favipiravir in the treatment of COVID-19. International Journal of Infectious Diseases. 2021;**102**:501-508

[21] Satarker S, Tom AA, Shaji RA, Alosious A, Luvis M, Nampoothiri M. JAK-STAT pathway inhibition and their implications in COVID-19 therapy. Postgraduate Medicine. 2020;**133**(5):1

[22] Jamilloux Y, el Jammal T, Vuitton L, Gerfaud-Valentin M, Kerever S, Sève P. JAK inhibitors for the treatment of autoimmune and inflammatory diseases. Autoimmunity Reviews. 2019;**18**(11)

[23] Levien TL, Baker DE. Remdesivir. Hospital Pharmacy. 2021. Available from: https://www.ncbi.nlm.nih.gov/books/NBK563261/

[24] Remdesivir—StatPearls. NCBI Bookshelf. Available from: https://www.ncbi.nlm.nih.gov/books/NBK563261/

[25] Coronavirus Disease (COVID-19): Dexamethasone. Available from: https://www.who.int/news-room/questions-and-answers/item/coronavirusdisease-covid-19-dexamethasone

[26] Paula HSC, Santiago SB, Araújo LA, Pedroso CF, Marinho TA, IAJ G, et al. An overview on the current available treatment for COVID-19 and the impact of antibiotic administration during the pandemic. Brazilian Journal of Medical and Biological Research. 2022;**55**

[27] Chari A, Vogl DT, Gavriatopoulou M, Nooka AK, Yee AJ, Huff CA, et al. Oral selinexor–dexamethasone for triple-class refractory multiple myeloma. New England Journal of Medicine;**381**(8):727-738

[28] Karyopharm to Evaluate Low Dose Selinexor as a Potential. Available from: https://www.globenewswire.com/news- release/2020/04/07/2012711/0/en/Karyopharm-to-Evaluate-Low-Dose-Selinexor-as-a-Potential-Treatment-for-Hospitalized-Patients-with-COVID-19.html

[29] Jayamohanan H, Venniyoor V, Pavithran K. Selinexor—A drug review. Indian Journal of Medical and Paediatric Oncology. 2021;**42**(4):360-363

[30] Selinexor: MedlinePlus Drug Information. Available from: https://medlineplus.gov/druginfo/meds/a619044.html

[31] Selinexor | C17H11F6N7O—PubChem. Available from: https://pubchem.ncbi.nlm.nih.gov/compound/Selinexor

[32] Fang W, Jiang J, Su L, Shu T, Liu H, Lai S, et al. The role of NO in COVID-19 and potential therapeutic strategies. Free Radical Biology and Medicine. 2021;**163**:153-162

[33] Nitric Oxide (Inhalation Route) Side Effects—Mayo Clinic. Available from: https://www.mayoclinic.org/drugs-supplements/nitric-oxide-inhalation-route/side-effects/drg-20060881?p=1

[34] Ichinose F, Roberts JD, Zapol WM. Inhaled nitric oxide: A selective pulmonary vasodilator: Current uses and therapeutic potential. Circulation;**109**(25):3106-3111. DOI: 10.1161/01.CIR.0000134595.80170.62

[35] Witek J. Nitric Oxide. ncbi.nlm.nih.gov 2020. Available from: https://www.ncbi.nlm.nih.gov/books/NBK554485/

[36] Ritonavir-Boosted Nirmatrelvir (Paxlovid) | COVID-19 Treatment Guidelines. Available from: https://www.covid19treatmentguidelines.nih.gov/therapies/antiviral-therapy/ritonavir-boosted-nirmatrelvir--paxlovid-/

[37] Coronavirus (COVID-19) Update: FDA Authorizes First Oral Antiviral for Treatment of COVID-19 | FDA. Available from: https://www.fda.gov/news-events/press-announcements/coronavirus-covid-19-update-fda-authorizes-first-oral-antiviral-treatment-covid-19

[38] 13 Things To Know About Paxlovid, the Latest COVID-19 Pill > News > Yale Medicine. Available from: https://www.yalemedicine.org/news/13-things-to-know-paxlovid-covid-19

[39] Is Paracetamol Effective in Treating or Curing COVID-19?. Available from: https://health-desk.org/articles/is-paracetamol-effective-in-treating-or-curing-covid-19

[40] Paracetamol for Adults: Painkiller to Treat Aches, Pains and Fever—NHS. Available from: https://www.nhs.uk/medicines/paracetamol-for-adults/

[41] Aranow C. Vitamin D and the immune system. Journal of investigative medicine: the official publication of the American Federation for Clinical Research. 2011;**59**(6):881-886

[42] Vitamin D | COVID-19 Treatment Guidelines. Available from: https://www.covid19treatmentguidelines.nih.gov/therapies/supplements/vitamin-d/

[43] Vitamin D: Overview, Uses, Side Effects, Precautions, Interactions, Dosing and Reviews. Available from: https://www.webmd.com/vitamins/ai/ingredientmono-929/vitamin-d

[44] Drisdol, Calciferol (vitamin D) Dosing, Indications, Interactions, Adverse Effects, and More. Available from: https://reference.medscape.com/drug/drisdol-calciferol-vitamind-344417

[45] Abobaker A, Alzwi A, Alraied AHA. Overview of the possible role of vitamin C in management of COVID-19. Pharmacological Reports. 2020;**72**(6):1517-1528. DOI: 10.1007/s43440-020-00176-1

[46] Vitamin C and COVID-19: A Review. Available from: https://www.news-medical.net/news/20201023/Vitamin-C-and-COVID-19-A-Review.aspx

[47] Vitamin C—Mayo Clinic. Available from: https://www.mayoclinic.org/drugs-supplements-vitamin-c/art-20363932

[48] Vitamins and Minerals—Vitamin C—NHS. Available from: https://www.nhs.uk/conditions/vitamins-and-minerals/vitamin-c/

[49] Zinc | The Nutrition Source | Harvard T.H. Chan School of Public Health. Available from: https://www.hsph.harvard.edu/nutritionsource/zinc/

[50] Kumar A, Kubota Y, Chernov M, Kasuya H. Potential role of zinc supplementation in prophylaxis and treatment of COVID-19. Medical Hypotheses. 2020;**144**:109848

[51] Zinc—Mayo Clinic. Available from: https://www.mayoclinic.org/drugs-supplements-zinc/art-20366112

[52] ZINC: Overview, Uses, Side Effects, Precautions, Interactions, Dosing and Reviews. Available from: https://www.webmd.com/vitamins/ai/ingredientmono-982/zinc

[53] Clinical Management Protocol For COVID-19 (In Adults) Government of India Ministry of Health and Family Welfare. Available from: https://www.mohfw.gov.in/pdf/UpdatedDetailedClinicalManagementProtocolforCOVID19adultsdated24052021.pdf

[54] WHO Coronavirus (COVID-19) Dashboard | WHO Coronavirus (COVID-19) Dashboard With Vaccination Data. Available from: https://covid19.who.int/

Chapter 7

COVID-19: From Pathophysiology to Treatment

Joise Wottrich, Eduardo Gonçalves, Carina Echer de Souza, Pauline Brendler Goettems Fiorin, Mirna Stela Ludwig, Thiago Gomes Heck and Matias Nunes Frizzo

Abstract

The new coronavirus first appeared in December 2019 in Wuhan, China, being officially named severe acute respiratory syndrome coronavirus 2 (SARS-CoV-2) by the International Committee on Taxonomy of Viruses (ICTV), as well as the name of the disease has been described as COVID-19 (coronavirus disease 2019). In March 2020, the disease was considered a global pandemic, with currently more than 514 million cases worldwide, with 6.4 million deaths. Severe cases of COVID-19 progress to acute respiratory distress syndrome (ARDS), on average about 8–9 days after the onset of symptoms. It is also worth mentioning that the severity of the disease in patients is not only due to the viral infection but also due to the host response. This phase, called a cytokine storm, reflects a state of systemic immune activation, with high levels of cytokines, such as IL-6, IL-1b, IL-2, IL-12, IL-18, TNF, and interferon gamma (IFN-γ). In this sense, the management of the disease largely depends on symptomatic and supportive treatments. For severely or critically ill patients with acute respiratory distress syndrome (ARDS) and sepsis, in addition to supplemental oxygen, mechanical ventilation, and ARDS-specific therapies, antiviral and antibiotic treatments should also be considered. Thus, the purpose of this chapter is to describe the pathophysiology and treatment of SARS-CoV-2 infection.

Keywords: SARS-CoV-2, COVID-19, pathophysiology, treatment

1. Introduction

Coronaviruses (CoVs) belong to the *order of Nidovirales, family of Coronaviridae, and* are divided into four genera: *alphacoronavirus, betacoronavirus, gammacoronavirus, and deltacoronavirus*. The term "Corona" is used because the virus has crown-like spikes on its external surface [1]. CoVs cause diseases in a wide variety of birds and mammals and have been found in humans since 1960. To date, seven human CoVs have been identified, including the alpha-CoVs HCoVs-NL63 and HCoVs-229E and the beta-CoVs HCoVs-OC43, HCoVs-HKU1, severe acute respiratory syndrome-CoV (SARS-CoV), and Middle East respiratory syndrome-CoV (MERS-CoV). The new coronavirus was first identified in December 2019 in Wuhan, China, being officially named by the International Committee on Virus Taxonomy (ICTV), as well as the name of the disease has been designated COVID-19 [2, 3].

SARS-CoV-2 is very contagious since it is able to spread easily from human to human through different routes of infection, such as droplets, contact, and aerosol transmission. Coronaviruses (CoVs) are the largest known RNA viruses, their size ranges from 65 to 125 nm in diameter, and their nucleic acid genome is a single-tape RNA, with a size ranging from 26 to 32 Kb. The CoVs HKU1, NL63, OC43, and 229E are associated with mild symptoms in humans, while SARS-CoV, MERS-CoV, and SARS-CoV-2, which belong to the genus betacoronavirus, cause severe pneumonia in humans [3].

CoVs were believed to infect only animals until an outbreak of severe acute respiratory syndrome (SARS) caused by SARS-CoV occurred in 2002 in Guangdong, China. A decade later, another pathogenic coronavirus, known as middle eastern respiratory syndrome coronavirus (MERS-CoV), caused an endemic disease in Middle Eastern countries. In late 2019, Wuhan, an emerging business center in China, experienced an outbreak of a new coronavirus that killed more than 1,800 people and infected more than 70,000 in the first fifty days of the epidemic. From the sequence-based analysis of isolates from patients, the virus was identified as a new coronavirus. In a recent review, it was demonstrated that the epicenter of the COVID-19 pandemic was similar to that of SARS-CoV-1, that is, a zoonotic origin. The most robust evidence points out that the Huanan market was the epicenter of the pandemic, probably the wildlife trade [4].

Because it is an RNA virus, SARS-CoV-2 presents a high mutation rate as its characteristic. This aspect provides conditions for this viral zoonotic pathogen to become more efficiently transmitted from person to person and possibly becoming more virulent. These observations indicated the ability of this virus to contaminate from human to human, which was subsequently reported worldwide [5]. In this sense, in March 2020, the disease was considered a global pandemic. Since then, there have been more than 575 million cases and 6.4 million deaths worldwide, according to data of the World Health Organization (WHO) in July 2022. In the same period, in Brazil, there were 33 million cases, with 679,000 deaths. The mortality rate in this country, according to the Brazilian Ministry of Health, is 32 people per 100,000 habitants.

Considering the epidemiological aspects of the pandemic, with emphasis on the mortality of COVID-19, disease therapy is a decisive tool in the conduction of patients and is fundamental for clinical improvement. Without specific treatment established for COVID-19 up to now, therapeutic support, such as the use of corticosteroids and oxygen supplementation, delivered the best results in large *trials.* In addition, interleukin blockers presented a good response in patients with the potential to progress to cytokine storm and acute respiratory distress syndrome (ARDS). Thus, the objective of this chapter is to describe the pathophysiology and treatment of SARS-CoV-2 infection, highlighting the importance of inflammatory biomarkers and knowledge of pathophysiology, and their interaction for early recognition of therapeutic targets (corticosteroids, oxygen supplementation), the need for hospitalization in intensive care units, as well as predict the evolution of the disease.

2. COVID-19

COVID-19 is a disease with high contagious power and clinical manifestations ranging from mild to severe, with the majority of the cases being mild. In current data, 81% of cases present mild symptoms and 1.2% are asymptomatic. The WHO estimates the reproductive number (R0) of SARS-CoV-2 between 2 and 2.5, which is higher than SARS (1.7–1.9) and MERS (<1), and demonstrates the highest pandemic potential of SARS-CoV-2. SARS-CoV-2 can spread rapidly in the community, unlike SARS-CoV and MERS-CoV, which have a higher mortality rate and a higher hospital admission rate [3]. Two main strains called "A" and "B" helped to track and know the viral genome of SARS-CoV-2, the difference between these two strains is only two nucleotides, and these characteristics are also found in coronavirus *of Rhinolophus*, the supposed host reservoir. Strain B has been the most common in the entire pandemic and includes all eleven sequenced human genomes directly associated with the Huanan market, The oldest human-line A genomes do not have a direct epidemiological connection with the Huanan market but have been identified in patients who have circulated in the vicinity of the market [6].

To enter host cells, SARS-CoV-2 shares the same human cell receptor with SARS-CoV, the angiotensin 2 converting enzyme (ACE-2), which is an ectoenzyme anchored in the plasma membrane of cells of various tissues, mainly in the lower respiratory tract, heart, kidneys, and gastrointestinal tract. The first critical step for the entry of the virus into sensitive host cells involves a specific receptor, usually, the CoVs enter the host cell using the transmembrane Spike glycoprotein (S). After the viral anchorage, transmembrane serine protease 2 (TMPRSS2) cleaves and activates the Spike protein: S1 binds to the receptor through its receptor-binding domain and S2 fuses the host membrane with the viral counterpart, an event that allows SARS-CoV-2 to enter the cells by endocytosis or direct fusion of the viral envelope with the host membrane [7].

Active replication and virus release cause the host cell to suffer pyroptosis and the discharge of pro-inflammatory chemical mediators, which are recognized by neighboring epithelial cells, endothelial cells, and alveolar macrophages, triggering the generation of pro-inflammatory and chemokine cytokines, including IL-6. Chemokines and pro-inflammatory cytokines attract monocytes, macrophages, and T cells to the site of infection, increasing the inflammatory picture (with the addition of IFNγ produced by T cells) and establishing a pro-inflammatory feedback cycle (**Figures 1** and **2**) [8].

In an impaired immune response, there may be a greater accumulation of immune cells in the lungs, causing overproduction of pro-inflammatory cytokines, which damages the lung infrastructure. The resulting cytokine storm circulates to other organs, promoting damage to various organs. In addition, non-neutralizing antibodies produced by B cells can increase SARS-CoV-2 infection through antibody-dependent enhancement, further exacerbating organ damage. Alternatively, in a healthy immune response, initial inflammation attracts virus-specific T cells to the site of infection, where they can eliminate infected cells before viral spread. Neutralizing antibodies in these individuals can block viral infection, and alveolar macrophages recognize neutralized viruses and apoptotic cells and eliminate them by phagocytosis, generating minimal inflammatory damage [8].

The mean incubation period of COVID-19 is 5 to 6 days, the mean age of COVID-19 cases ranges from 49 to 57 years, and the mean time from the first symptom to death is 14 days. Within 5 to 6 days of the onset of symptoms, the viral load of SARS-CoV-2 reaches its peak, being significantly earlier than that of SARS-CoV, in which the period of viral load peak is about 10 days after the onset of symptoms [9].

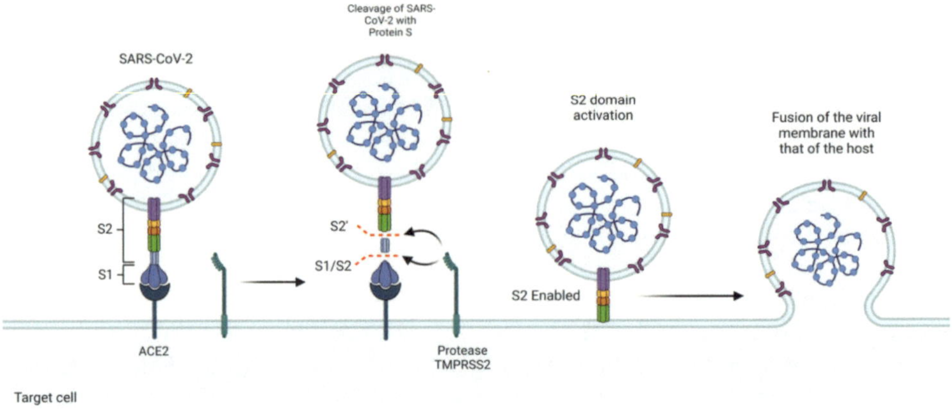

Figure 1.
Connection of SARS-CoV-2 to ACE-2 receptors. Figure describes: The connection of SARS-Cov-2 with the ACE2 receptor on the target cell, followed by cleavage of SARS-CoV-2 with the S protein, activation of the S2 domain, and fusion of the viral membrane with the host cell. Source: Figure of the authors.

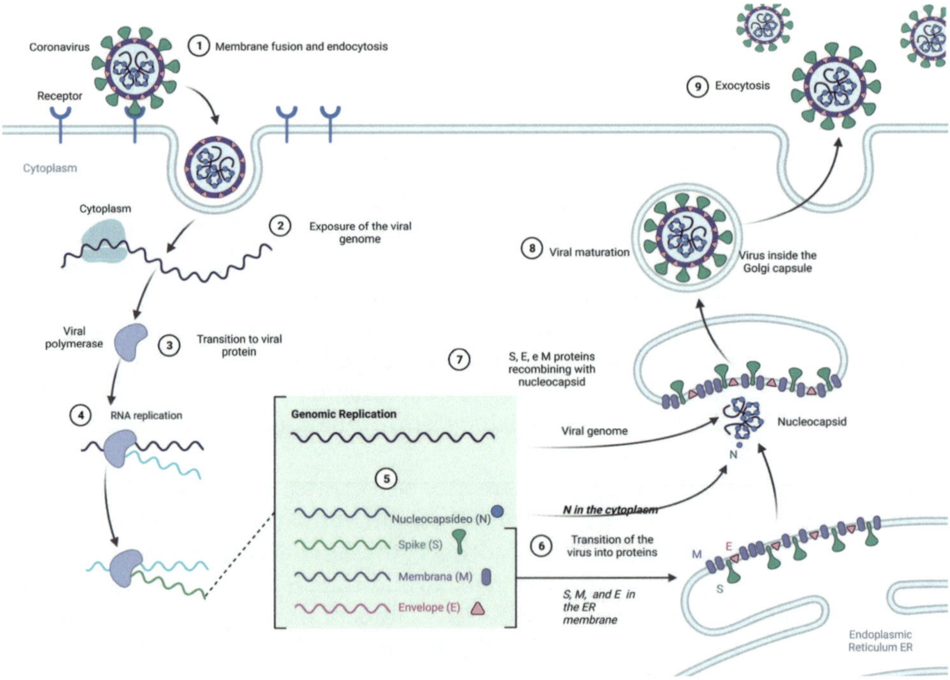

Figure 2.
Viral replication of SARS-CoV-2. Figure describes: 1) Fusion of the virus to the host membrane, occurring endocytosis; 2) Exposure of the viral genome; 3) viral polymerase performs transcription for viral protein; 4) viral replication occurs; 5) genomic replication; 6) transition of the virus into proteins in the membrane of the endoplasmic reticulum; 7) proteins S, E, and M recombining with nucleocapsid; 8) viruses within the Golgi capsule, performing viral maturation; and 9) viral exocytosis. Source: Figure of the authors.

Severe cases of COVID-19 progress to acute respiratory distress syndrome (ARDS), on average, about 8–9 days after the onset of symptoms. It is also worth mentioning that the severity of the disease in patients is not only due to viral infection but also due to the response of the host [8], as shown in **Figures 3** and **4**.

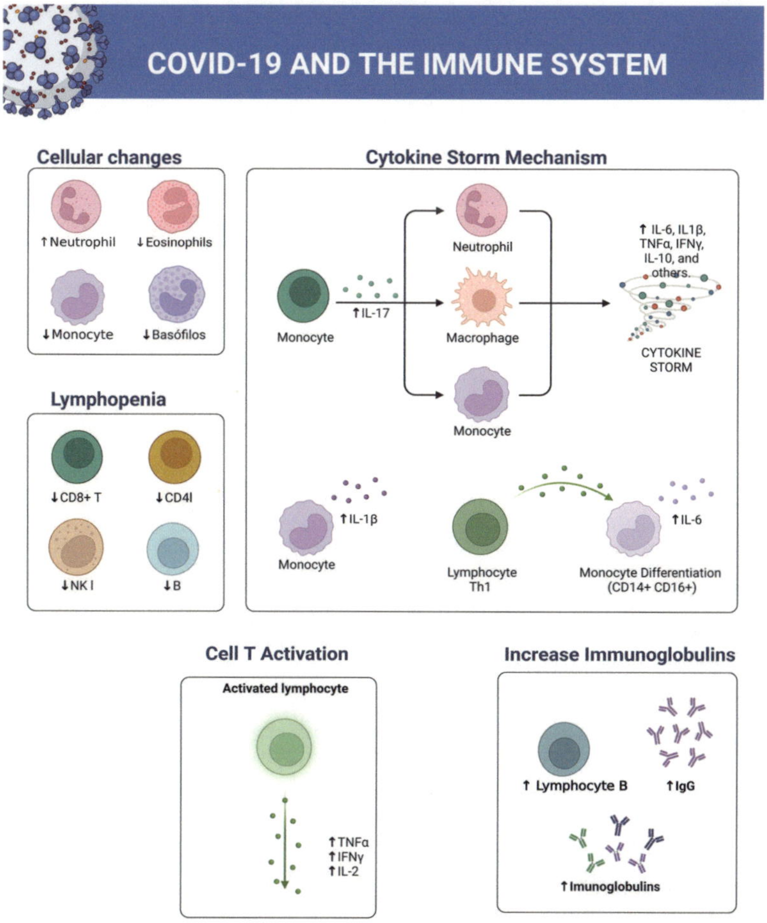

Figure 3.
Innate and adaptive immune response at COVID-19. Description of the most frequent cellular alterations in COVID-19: increase of neutrophils and decrease of eosinophils, monocytes, and basophils. Lymphopenia occurs due to a decrease in CD4, Cd8, B and natural killer lymphocytes. The activated T lymphocyte promotes the increase of TNF, Interferon, and IL-2. The activation of B lymphocytes promotes the increase of immunoglobulins G. In the storm of cytokines occurs an uncontrolled elevation of IL-6, IL-1, TNF, interferon gamma, and IL-10. Source: Figure of the authors.

SARS-CoV-2 infection in severe cases leads to activation of macrophages and dendritic cells and consequent exacerbated release of pro-inflammatory cytokines. In addition, the presentation of SARS-CoV-2 antigens through the main histocompatibility complexes I and II (MHC I and II) stimulates humoral and cellular immunity, also resulting in the high production of cytokines. When the virus reaches the lower respiratory tract and infects type II pneumocytes, it promotes apoptosis and loss of surfactant, capillary extravasation, and alveolar edema, resulting in lung damage and collapse, impairing gas exchange [10].

The onset and duration of the cytokine storm vary, depending on the cause and treatments administered. Most patients with cytokine storm present fever, fatigue, anorexia, headache, rash, diarrhea, arthralgia, myalgia, and neuropsychiatric findings. These symptoms may be directly due to cytokine-induced tissue damage or acute phase physiological changes or may result from immune cell-mediated responses. Cases may progress rapidly to disseminated intravascular coagulation with vascular

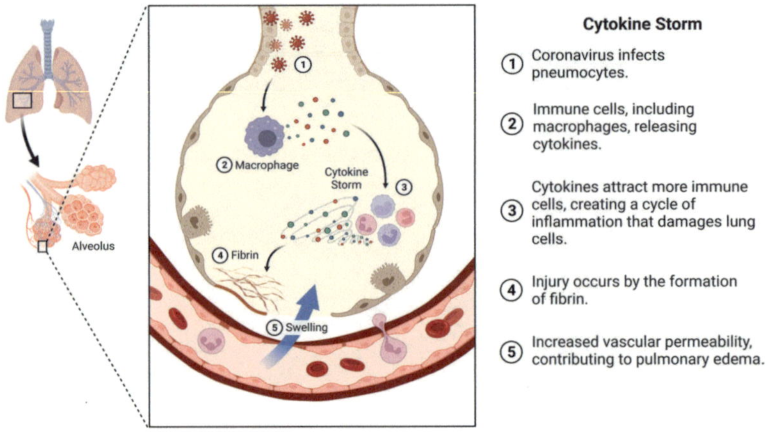

Figure 4.
Cytokine storm at COVID-19. Description of the pathophysiology of cytokine storm, after the entry of the virus into the pneumocyte, occurs activation of macrophages with the release of cytokines, generating damage to lung cells, with fibrin formation, increased vascular permeability, and pulmonary edema. Source: Figure of the authors.

occlusion or catastrophic hemorrhage, dyspnea, hypoxemia, hypotension, hemostatic imbalance, septic shock, and death [11].

Since the initial phase of the pandemic, the cytokine storm has become peculiar to SARS-COV-2 infection, at least in severe cases. It is responsible for damaging the respiratory tract and subsequent failure of multiple organs. It results from a complex network involving cytokines/chemokines/infiltrating immune cells that orchestrate the aberrant immune response in COVID-19. This term covers several disorders of immune dysregulation and is characterized by constitutional symptoms, systemic inflammation, and multiple organ dysfunction [12].

The combination of hyperinflammation, coagulopathy, and low platelet count puts patients with cytokine storm at high risk of spontaneous bleeding. Among the most commonly described biomarkers are interleukin I 1β, IL-6, tumor necrosis factor (TNF) α, interferon (IFN) γ, and IL-10. The cytokine storm sustains too much inflammatory response in the blood, causing the immune system to attack the body involving various organs, such as the lungs. This, in turn, causes injury to the alveolar-capillary membrane, increased pulmonary permeability, acute respiratory distress syndrome, and multiple organ failure [13].

In the pathophysiology of cytokine storm, we can highlight macrophage activation, a hyperinflammatory condition associated with different triggers, including infections, autoimmune diseases, and neoplasms, being characterized by fever, hepatosplenomegaly, cytopenias, elevated levels of ferritin, triglycerides, lactic dehydrogenase, D-dimer and aminotransferases, as well as hypofibrinogenemia. The acute phase of the syndrome reflects a state of systemic immune activation, with elevated cytokine levels such as IL-6, IL-1b, IL-2, IL-12, IL-18, TNF, and interferon gamma (IFN-γ). The term macrophage activation syndrome (AMS) refers to a subgroup of patients with secondary hemophagocytic lymphohistiocytosis, in a context of self-ignition or systemic autoimmunity, characterized by hyperinflammatory and hyperferritinemic immune responses, directed by different T lymphocyte subpopulations and associated with cytokine release syndrome [9], as illustrated in **Figure 4**.

3. Treatment of COVID-19

To date, no pharmacological intervention has been shown to be effective and safe to ensure its use in the routine treatment of patients with COVID-19; therefore, ideally, these patients have been treated in the context of clinical trials and guidelines for good clinical practice. In newly emerging diseases, such as COVID-19, especially in a pandemic situation, interventions are mainly performed *based on in vitro experiments, personal experiments,* and small limited observational studies. The management of the disease depends largely on symptomatic and supportive treatments [14].

Worldwide, several pharmacological interventions have been proposed for COVID-19, such as anticoagulants, antimicrobials, chloroquine, hydroxychloroquine, convalescent plasma, remdesivir, and tocilizumab [14]. For severely or critically ill patients with acute respiratory distress syndrome (ARDS) and sepsis, in addition to supplemental oxygen, mechanical ventilation and specific therapies for ARDS, antiviral and antibiotic treatments should also be considered [15, 16].

3.1 Steroids

The use of systemic corticosteroid therapy in the treatment of infectious diseases is controversial, however, widely used. Corticosteroids have received worldwide attention as a potentially effective treatment for COVID-19 infection [15]. In the COVID-19 Randomized Trial of Therapy (RECOVERY), the use of dexamethasone resulted in lower mortality rates in individuals with COVID-19 who received mechanical ventilation or supplemental oxygen [17]. In the CoDEX study in patients with COVID-19 and moderate or severe ARDS, the use of dexamethasone resulted in a statistically significant increase in the number of days without mechanical ventilation, but without impact on mortality [18].

Pathologies that present an increase in endogenous levels of glucocorticoids (CG) are sepsis, cachexia, metabolic acidosis, and severe insulinopenia. GC-induced muscle atrophy is characterized by rapidly contracting glycolytic muscle atrophy, decreased fiber cross-sectional area, and reduced myofibrillar protein content [19, 20]. Glucocorticoids lead to an imbalance between the rate of synthesis and degradation of proteins. Dexamethasone, a synthetic glucocorticoid, stimulates skeletal muscle atrophy by promoting protein degradation [19] through the ubiquitin-proteasome pathways and by inhibiting protein synthesis via Akt/(mTOR) [21].

According to Shang et al. [22], patients with COVID-19 release elevated cytokine levels, showing that alveolar damage is steroid-responsive. The RECOVERY study established that dexamethasone can significantly decrease mortality in severe cases of COVID-19, especially in critical conditions when ventilatory support is necessary, presumably because the severity of lung injury reflects worsening of the hyperinflammation. The reason for dexamethasone to be chosen included its anti-inflammatory potency, lack of mineralocorticoid effect, and longer action profile [23]. Pharmacological responses require exposure to high doses of corticosteroids, *and in vitro studies have shown* a higher response with methylprednisolone than with dexamethasone [24], and this preference is sustained when the inflammatory pathway and characteristics of the different corticosteroids are considered. In addition, treatment with methylprednisolone for a shorter period may also minimize systemic side effects [25]. The trial of Ko et al. [26], provided evidence that the mortality benefit of dexamethasone in severe COVID-19 is not drug-specific but rather the general anti-inflammatory effect of corticosteroids. In this study, the higher anti-inflammatory potency of methylprednisolone showed additional mortality benefits, especially in patients who required mechanical ventilation.

The Brazilian guideline for the pharmacological treatment of hospitalized patients reviewed several studies worldwide, bringing a strong recommendation for the use of dexamethasone (6 mg/day for 10 days) only in individuals who are under the use of supplemental oxygen therapy since at the Brazilian level, this drug has good tolerance on the part of the patient and low cost for health institutions. There is no evidence for the use of routine corticosteroids in patients with COVID-19, especially, this should still be avoided within the first 7 to 10 days of the onset of the symptoms, when the host response is fighting the viral infection. Some evidence suggests retardation in viral clearance when corticosteroids are used early. The potential benefit of its use would be in patients with moderate to severe ARDS, in selected cases and without suspicion of uncontrolled bacterial infection, 10–14 days after the onset of COVID-19 symptoms. The doses used in the studies ranged from 10 mg to 20 mg of dexamethasone and 40 mg to 120 mg of methylprednisolone per day for 5–10 days [14].

The Brazilian recommendation is in accordance with the WHO guideline Corticosteroids for COVID-19 launched in September 2020, which reviewed meta-analyses and randomized trials with data from more than 7,000 patients. The WHO panel recommends the use of oral or intravenous glucocorticoids for 7 to 10 days in patients with severe and critical COVID-19, defined by the presence of signs of respiratory distress, increase in respiratory rate, hypoxemia, necessity of vasopressor therapy, and/or mechanical ventilation, regardless of their hospitalization status. The recommendation is supported by evidence of 6.7 to 8.7% reduction in 28-day mortality and reduction in the need for invasive mechanical ventilation. Different GC can be selected, according to availability and observing equivalent doses. The daily dose of 6 mg of dexamethasone is equivalent to 40 mg of prednisone, 160 mg of hydrocortisone (e.g., 50 mg every 8 hours or 100 mg every 12 hours), or 32 mg of methylprednisolone (e.g., 8 mg every 6 hours or 16 mg every 12 hours). The panel also recommends to monitor glucose levels and other potential GC adverse effects, and not to use GC in non-severe COVID-19, due to a potential risk of increasing death in this setting. One should also adjudicate the risk of secondary and endemic infections and act to minimize their risk.

An important aspect to consider is that the increase in cortisol and bed rest act synergistically on the decrease in muscle mass. It has been demonstrated that after 28 days, healthy young individuals lost more muscles when confined to bed and received hydrocortisone than only at rest [27]. The restriction of movements during hospitalization of COVID-19 in the ICU is different from other clinical conditions, because the patient with COVID-19 may present deep weakness, spend hours on high-flow oxygen therapy or in ventral decubitus. A median reduction of 18.5% of the rectus femoris muscle between the first and seventh day of ICU stay may occur [28]. In addition, the study by Kirwan et al. [29] demonstrated an unadjusted risk of sarcopenia of 38.4% associated with an average time of 11 days in hospital stay by COVID-19.

One of the main side effects of GC use is hyperglycemia, and this condition is also induced by the course of critical disease [30]. The diabetogenic effect of steroids in susceptible patients can aggravate the problem of anabolic resistance. The hyperglycemia of the critically ill patient is related to insulin resistance, that is, the impossibility of insulin to stimulate glucose uptake in skeletal muscle or to inhibit gluconeogenesis in the liver. During critical disease, the abrupt development of hyperglycemia involves complex interactions between some counterregulatory hormones (glucagon, catecholamines, growth hormone, and cortisol), adipokines, and inflammatory cytokines that cause increased glucose production by the liver and insulin resistance in tissues. This hyperglycemia can affect the functions of respiratory muscles, leading to respiratory muscle weakness acquired in the ICU, as well as increase mortality in these patients [5]. Insulin resistance ultimately promotes a catabolic state that implies lipolysis and loss of muscle mass [31].

3.2 IL-6 antagonists

Tocilizumab is an interleukin 6 inhibitor approved for the treatment of rheumatoid arthritis, giant cell arteritis, and cytokine release syndrome during chimeric antigen receptor (CAR-T) T-cell therapy. Interleukin 6 is an inflammatory cytokine that exerts its effects on the liver and lymphocytes, inducing acute phase reagents such as C-reactive protein, fibrinogen, and hepatocytes hepcidin, and promotes the differentiation of cytotoxic T cells CD4 (T helper 17) and CD8 and antibody production. Interleukin 6 plays an important role in controlling viral infections such as influenza A, acute severe respiratory syndrome coronavirus 1, and herpes virus. In COVID-19, an increased level of interleukin 6 and C-reactive protein correlates with the severity and mortality of the disease. Thus, blocking the activity of interleukin 6 may play a role in mitigating the inflammatory response and improving clinical outcomes in patients with COVID-19 [32].

The World Health Organization's (WHO) Rapid Evidence Assessment Working Group (REACT) developed a protocol to perform a prospective meta-analysis of IL-6 antagonists in patients hospitalized by COVID-19. The IL-6 antagonists investigated were monoclonal antibodies that bind to soluble, membrane-bound IL-6 receptors (e.g., tocilizumab and sarilumab) or directly to IL-6 (e.g., siltuximab). Administration of IL-6 antagonists, compared to usual treatment or placebo, was associated with lower all-cause mortality in 28 days [33]. Tocilizumab is a humanized antibody against IL-6 and has been used in patients with pronounced cytokine storm. Patients with rheumatoid arthritis who regularly use this medication have demonstrated that long-term treatment with tocilizumab leads to increased muscle mass, as assessed with *dual X-ray absorptiometry* (DEXA) [34]. Tocilizumab reduces the risk of mechanical ventilation in hospitalized patients [35] and also reduces all-cause mortality on day 28 compared to standard treatment alone or with placebo [36] (**Figure 5**).

According to the available studies [17, 37], tocilizumab was recommended by Brazilian treatment guidelines for patients with COVID-19, who are using NIV (non-invasive mechanical ventilation) or CNAF (high flow nasal catheter) and not recommended in patients under mechanical ventilation. To date, the studies have not shown clear benefits in patients under mechanical ventilation; however, there is a tendency to prescribe it in the first 24 hours of IMV, at medical discretion. However, the authors indicate that the package leaflet of this medicine does not present this indication [28], that is, its use in MV *would be off-label,* and access to this drug may be limited by availability and also financial reasons.

The indicated dosage is 8 mg/kg, with a maximum administration of 800 mg, and a second application should only be performed after careful medical reassessment. Evidence also suggests that the benefits of tocilizumab are associated with corticosteroid co-administration [17] and may preferably be used in patients with increased inflammatory markers (C-reactive protein test, ferritin, and lactic dehydrogenase).

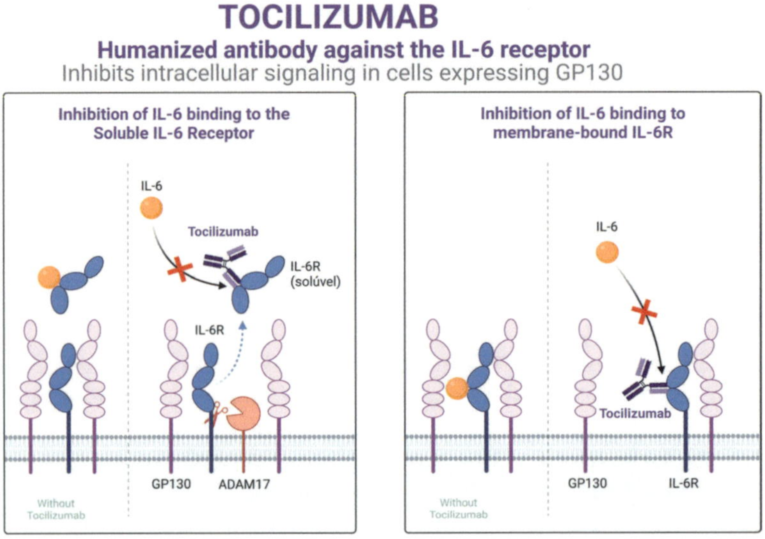

Figure 5.
Tocilizumab mechanism of action. Tocilizumab is a recombinant humanized monoclonal antibody, which acts as an interleukin 6 receptor antagonist (IL-6), blocking the transduction of the signal of this pro-inflammatory cytokine, preventing the dimerization of GP130 in the cell membrane and, consequently, blocks the proinflammatory effects of IL-6. In addition, it has the ability to dissociate IL-6/IL-6R complexes that have already formed. The IL-6 receptor has two presentations: membrane-bound IL-6 receptor and soluble IL-6 receptor. IL-6 is binding with IL-6R for the formation of a complex, which is coupled to the transmembrane protein gp130 so that signal transduction occurs and pro-inflammatory function is performed. Source: Figure of the authors.

For patients with signs of bacterial infection, with latent infections such as tuberculosis or parasitic, care should be given to the possibility of reactivation of these with the administration of tocilizumab. In immunosuppressed patients, its use should be with caution, and in neutropenic individuals (<500 cells/mm^3), thrombocytopenic (< 50,000 platelets/mm^3) or with transaminases at levels five times greater than physiological value, tocilizumab should not be used at all [14].

In addition to tocilizumab, other trials that use Casirivimab and Imdevimab are presenting significantly promising results, however, only in patients in the early stages of the disease [38, 39] and not in hospitalized patients. Recommendations of the treatment panel for COVID-19 for the treatment of outpatients, by order of preference, are nirmatrelvir enhanced with ritonavir (Paxlovid) (AIIa) and remdesivir (BIIa). Other alternative medicines, such as Bebtelovimab (CIII) and Molnupiravir (IIC), should be used only when none of the first-rate medicines are available.

It is also worth noting that the treatments with antiviral drugs that the WHO panel against indicates are interferons for outpatients (AIIa), interferon alpha or lambda for hospitalized patients (AIIa), Ivermectin (AIIa), Nitazoxanide (BIIa), Chloroquine or hydroxychloroquine and/or azithromycin for hospitalization (AI) and not hospitalization situation (AIIa), Lopinavir/ritonavir and other HIV protease inhibitors for hospitalized patients (AI) and outpatients (AIII) and systemic interferon beta for hospitalized patients (AI). Due to these concerns and data gaps, Molnupiravir should be provided only to non-severe patients with COVID-19 at higher risk of hospitalization. Typically, they are people who have not received COVID-19 vaccination, elderly people with immunodeficiencies or people living with chronic diseases.

Treatment with anti-SARS-CoV-2 mAbs should be considered for patients with mild-to-moderate COVID-19 who are hospitalized, considering that the risk of progression to severe COVID-19 in high-risk patients is substantially higher for those who are not vaccinated. It is also interesting to note that severely immunocompromised patients may have prolonged replication of SARS-CoV-2, leading to faster viral evolution, with consequent worse clinical outcomes. Anti-SARS-CoV-2 monoclonal antibodies (mAbs) have their results variable, depending on the circulating strain. As a suggestion, the use of anti-SARS-CoV-2 mAbs is based on current knowledge of SARS-CoV-2 in vitro activities. At the moment, the recommendations of the panel's anti-SARS-CoV-2 mAb are for the treatment of patients with mild-to-moderate COVID-19 who are at high risk of progressing to severe disease.

Intravenous Bebtelovimab has its use only for patients aged ≥12 years as an alternative therapy when nirmatrelvir (Paxlovid) and remdesivir potentiated with ritonavir are not available, viable to use, or clinically appropriate (CIII). Treatment should be started as soon as possible and within 7 days after the onset of symptoms. Anti-SARS-CoV-2 mAbs should be administered in an environment where severe hypersensitivity reactions such as anaphylaxis can be controlled. Patients should be monitored during the infusion and observed for at least 1 hour after infusion.

3.3 Anticoagulants

The care team should pay attention to the development of signs and symptoms of thromboembolic events. Due to this risk, patients hospitalized due to COVID-19 should receive prophylaxis of thromboembolism according to their risk stratification, according to current hospital protocols, for presenting in a high state of hypercoagulability, with a high rate of thromboembolic events being observed in observational and postmortem clinical studies. The dose to be used may vary according to the chosen class, for example, enoxaparin 40 to 60 mg SC once a day or the unfractionated heparin 5,000IU SC two to three times a day. Although evidence for pharmacological prophylaxis in the context of COVID-19 is limited, the intervention is low cost and well-tolerated, with the potential to avoid events of high clinical importance. Heparin should not be used in the case of contraindications of high risk of bleeding, active bleeding, and severe thrombocytopenia [40].

Critically ill patients have a strong recommendation for prophylactic doses for venous thromboembolism with anticoagulant (mainly with the use of vasoactive drugs, on hemodialysis or using CNAF, NIV, or MV), according to the Brazilian guidelines for pharmacological treatment for COVID-19. But there is no recommendation for the use of intermediate doses in patients without signs of thromboembolism. Anticoagulants should be used, following a careful assessment of bleeding risk and presence of thrombocytopenias [14].

In a study evaluating 42 patients, all using immunosuppressant or glucocorticosteroids, with severe to moderate COVID-19, with 21 patients receiving low-molecular weight heparin and 21 controls, there was a significant reduction. In IL-6 dosage and increased lymphocytes. The results of this study contribute to the use of low-molecular weight heparin as a potential therapeutic drug for the treatment of COVID-19. Changes in D-dimer levels and fibrinogen degradation products in the group that received heparin before and after treatment were significantly different from those in the control group ($P = 0.035$). Together, IL-6 levels have also been reduced after heparin treatment ($P = 0.006$), indicating that, in addition to other beneficial properties, it can exert an anti-inflammatory effect and partly attenuate the virus-induced "cytokine storm" [41].

There is no indication of routine use of anticoagulants in post-discharge due to COVID-19. The indication of the use of anticoagulants in a post-discharge setting should follow the same criteria as for patients without COVID-19, according to institutional protocols.

3.4 Antimicrobials (antibiotics)

Patients with COVID-19 without signs of sepsis or infection are not recommended for antibiotic therapy. However, individuals who present potential infectious foci on admission, with suspected sepsis, presenting or not being diagnosed for COVID-19, are indicated for the use of antibiotics (empirically). Also, patients with worsening due to COVID-19, who require care in intensive care units, are exposed to processes that potentiate the risk of infection, such as mechanical ventilation, bladder catheter, and arterial and venous accesses, which can lead to the need for the use of antibiotic therapy to this population [14].

To date, there is no randomized clinical trial evaluating the effectiveness of empirical antibacterials in patients with COVID-19 without evidence of bacterial infection, that is, clinical data are insufficient to demonstrate benefits or risks in the use of antibacterials in patients with COVID-19 without evidence of bacterial infection, so in the absence of evidence, there is no basis to indicate prophylactic antibacterials in patients with COVID-19. In addition to the absence of evidence of benefit, this practice may result in adverse events, increased antimicrobial resistance, and costs. There are no adequate data on bacterial co-infection in patients with COVID-19; however, it should be noted that the overlap of infections is possible to occur, mainly due to immunosuppression and exposure to the hospital environment, often colonized by multidrug-resistant germs. It is understood that these patients should receive antibacterials in a similar way to patients without COVID-19, following local protocols.

In the meta-analysis of Lanford [42] with 3,338 eligible patients, bacterial co-infection (estimated at presentation) was identified in 3.5% of patients (95% CI 0.4–6.7%) and secondary bacterial infection in 14.3% of patients (95% CI 9.6–18.9%). The overall proportion of patients with COVID-19 with bacterial infection was 6.9% (95% CI 4.3–9.5%). Bacterial infection was more common in critically ill patients (8.1%, 95% CI 2.3–13.8%). Since bacterial co-infection is relatively infrequent in patients hospitalized with COVID-19, therefore, most of these patients may not require empirical antibacterial treatment, reinforcing the guidelines of following institutional protocols for sepsis.

3.5 Oxygen therapy

Lung injury due to the new coronavirus resembles other causes of ARDS, but initial clinical features include more evident hypoxemia and loss of dyspnea perception. Due to the various forms of presentation of COVID-19, oxygen supplementation levels may vary according to clinical and laboratory signs. According to Guan [9], almost half (42%) of patients admitted to the hospital environment will require supplemental oxygen therapy. Nationwide, in the first five months of the pandemic, 49% of those infected required noninvasive respiratory support [43].

Oxygen therapy is defined as oxygen therapy, the administration of oxygen above the ambient air concentration (~21%), aiming to maintain adequate oxygenation of tissues. Its use has the potential to correct hypoxemia by reducing cardiorespiratory work overload [18]. Therefore, oxygen therapy is one of the treatments for the clinical condition in more severe cases of SARS-CoV-2 infection, since patients presenting hypoxemia or signs of respiratory effort may benefit from its use, either via the ocular nasal catheter, mask with a non-rebreathing oxygen mask, noninvasive ventilation (NIV), or high-flow nasal catheter (HFNC) [44]. If there is a need for oxygen therapy, it is recommended to be given its administration according to peripheral oxygen saturation (SpO2), with a strong recommendation of its onset when SpO2 <90%, in order to keep it between 92% and 96% in previously healthy patients and between 88% and 92% for patients with chronic lung disease [45].

3.5.1 High flow nasal cannula – HFNC

Prior to the COVID-19 pandemic, HFNC was already recommended in patients with moderate respiratory failure [46] and demonstrated efficacy in the treatment of acute hypercapnic respiratory failure [47, 48]. In CNAF, the supplementary supply of oxygen allows the administration of high flows (up to 60 liters per minute) and precise oxygen concentrations (21% to 100%) [49]. Even if there is no routine recommendation, when HFNC is indicated, it can be used in selected patients with hypoxemic respiratory failure associated with COVID-19, who have clinical signs and symptoms such as SpO2 < 93%, PaO2/FiO2 <300 mmHg, and respiratory rate > 25 incursions per minute [50].

3.5.2 Noninvasive mechanical ventilation – NIV

NIV contributes to the improvement of oxygenation and reduction of respiratory work and may prevent orotracheal intubation [51]. In viral pandemic disease, NIV has no recommendations for the treatment of hypoxemic respiratory failure [52], and depending on the interface used, large aerosol dispersion (COVID-19 dissemination medium) [53] can occur, so its indication should be judicious, and its application should be closely monitored.

The success of NIV to avoid intubation seems to be associated with patients with PaO2/FiO2 ratio > 100 mmHg and without multiple organ failure (APACHE < 20 score). During the first 30 minutes, ventilometry monitoring is very important, because a minute volume > 10l/min, current volume > 9 ml/kg predicted, respiratory rate > 25 irpm, requiring final expiratory positive pressure > 10 cmH20 with FiO2 > 50%, indicate its failure [50, 54].

3.5.3 Invasive mechanical ventilation – IMV

Among individuals infected with SARS-CoV-2, approximately 80% of the cases are asymptomatic, 15% present a more severe form (requiring supplemental oxygen), and 5% evolve to the most critical form, requiring advanced life support [41, 44]. This can occur mainly in patients with chronic heart or lung diseases, diabetes, obesity (BMI > 40), and in the elderly [51]. A recent study with biopsy of the diaphragm muscle showed the expression of ECA 2 and viral infiltration SARS-CoV-2 in the diaphragm of a subset of patients and histological evidence for the development of fibrosis [41].

The findings in the severe form of COVID-19 meet the diagnostic criteria for ARDS [55], and when hypoxemia worsens, hypercapnia, acidemia, respiratory fatigue, hemodynamic instability, or even mental status alterations, intubation should be strongly considered [50, 56], consequently requiring invasive mechanical ventilation (IMV). For those who need IMV, the objectives of this therapy are based on: maintenance of gas exchange (by correction of hypoxemia and respiratory acidosis associated with hypercapnia), reduction of respiratory work (with reversal or prevention of fatigue of respiratory muscles), and application of other specific and necessary treatment routes [57].

The long-term prognosis of patients who survive intensive care is affected by physical disabilities, cognitive impairments, and mental disorders that may occur after discharge from the ICU [58]. In relation to muscle mass loss, it may occur more frequently in older adults and patients with comorbidities who are more likely to have pre-existing catabolism. In addition, these groups of patients may be prone to develop more intense catabolic responses due to COVID-19 and prolonged ICU stay [59].

In addition to the systemic inflammatory process with cytokine release that contributes to the evolution of ARDS in critically ill patients with COVID-19, these patients also have an increased risk for weakness and sarcopenia due to the same inflammatory mechanism of loss of muscle mass. Associated with these factors, the length of stay on mechanical ventilation is high (mean of 11.7 days). About 75%–80% of patients hospitalized with COVID-19 have extended hospital stays, with about 21 days. When admitted to the ICU, they may have multiple organ failures, including ARDS, acute kidney injury, heart injury, and liver dysfunction [60]. Evidence has shown that organic dysfunction is highly associated with muscle dysfunction [61]. Additionally, some of these patients have associated comorbidities, such as advanced age, renal dysfunction, hypertension, diabetes, and heart disease, which may contribute to the incidence of weakness and sarcopenia. Thus, critical patients with COVID-19 may face a vicious cycle, in which the severity of the disease itself, the presence of comorbidities, prolonged invasive ventilatory support, and the use of sedatives and neuromuscular blockers may contribute to the development of weakness, sarcopenia, and functional dysfunctions in the short and long term [60].

4. Final considerations

Research and science are essential for the successful conduction of the COVID-19 pandemic. In this context, discovering the entry mechanism of the virus into a cell, the expected response of the host, and especially the exacerbated response in the form of the cytokine storm were fundamental for the initiation of clinical reasoning of diagnostic and therapeutic approaches. The unfavorable evolution of the clinical presentation of COVID-19 has led and still leads countless patients to need treatment in the intensive care unit (ICU), and sarcopenia and secondary infectious processes are a potential risk for the worsening of the clinical outcome [42, 62–87].

Thus, the intense scientific and technological advances in recent years of this pandemic favored the understanding and elucidation of the pathophysiology of the disease, and this knowledge is a crucial point for the use of existing drugs, such as tocilizumab, for the development of promising drugs and application of assistance protocols. The application of biomarkers, both clinical and laboratory, is differential when managing COVID-19, especially to stratify risk groups, monitor evolution, make therapeutic decisions, and in prognosis.

DOI: http://dx.doi.org/10.5772/intechopen.107146

Author details

Joise Wottrich[1*], Eduardo Gonçalves[2], Carina Echer de Souza[3], Pauline Brendler Goettems Fiorin[1], Mirna Stela Ludwig[1], Thiago Gomes Heck[1] and Matias Nunes Frizzo[1]

1 Regional University of the Northwest of the State of Rio Grande do Sul, Brazil

2 Brazilian Association of Cardiorespiratory Physiotherapy and Intensive Care Physiotherapy, Brazil

3 Oncology Institute of Ijui, Brazil

*Address all correspondence to: joise.wottrich@sou.unijui.edu.br

References

[1] Shereen MA, Khan S, Kazmi A, et al. COVID-19 infection: Emergence, transmission and characteristics of human coronavirus. Journal of Advanced Research. 2020;**24**:91

[2] COVID-19 Treatment Guidelines Panel. Coronavirus Disease 2019 (COVID-19) Treatment Guidelines. 2019. National Institutes of Health. Available from: https://www. covid19treatmentguidelines. nih.gov/ [Accessed: August 2, 2022]

[3] Bchetnia M, Girard C, Duchaine C, et al. The outbreak of the new acute severe respiratory syndrome coronavirus 2 (SARS-CoV-2): A review of the current global status. Journal of Infection and Public Health. 2020;**13**(11):1601-1610

[4] Worobey M et al. The Huanan Seafood Wholesale Market in Wuhan was the early epicenter of the COVID-19 pandemic. Science. 2022;**87**:8715

[5] Wang C, Horby PW, Hayden FG, et al. A new outbreak of coronavirus of global health concern. The Lancet, [S.L.] (Elsevier BV). Feb 2020;**395**(10223):470-473. DOI: 10.1016/s0140-6736(20)30185-9. Available from: https://www.thelancet.com/journals/lancet/article/PIIS0140-6736(20)30185-9/fulltext [Accessed: 10 May, 2021]

[6] Pekar JE et al. The molecular epidemiology of multiple zoonotic origins of SARS-CoV-2. Science. 2022;**83**:37

[7] Romano M, Ruggiero A, Squeglia F, et al. A structural view of the SARS-CoV-2 RNA replication machine: RNA synthesis, revision and final capping. Cells. 2020;**9**:1267

[8] Tay MZ, Poh CM, Rénia L, et al. The trinity of COVID-19: Immunity, inflammation and intervention. Nature Reviews Imunology. 2020;**20**:363

[9] Guan WJ, Ni ZY, Hu Y, et al. Clinical features of coronavirus disease 2019 in China. New England Journal of Medicine. 2021;**382**(18):1708

[10] Rabi FA, Zoubi MSA, Kasasbeh GA, et al. SARS-CoV-2 and Coronavirus Disease 2019: What we know so far. Pathogens. 2020;**9**:231

[11] Fajgenbaum DC, June CH. Cytokine storm. New England Journal of Medicine. 2021;**383**(23):2255-2273

[12] Coperchini F, Chiovato L, Rotondi M. Interleukin-6, CXCL10 and infiltrating macrophages in COVID-19-related cytokine storm: Not one for everyone, but for all for one! Borders in Immunology. 2021;**12**:1-8

[13] Xiong F, Tang H, Liu L, et al. Clinical features and medical interventions for COVID-19 in Hemodialysis Patients in Wuhan, China. JASN. 2020;**31**:1387

[14] Falavigna M, Stein C, Amaral JLG, et al. Brazilian guidelines for the pharmacological treatment of patients hospitalized with COVID-19. Rev Bras Have Intensive. 2022;**34**(1):1-12

[15] Sanders JM, Monogue ML, Jodlowski TZ, Cutrell JB. Pharmacologic treatments for coronavirus disease 2019 (COVID-19): A review. JAMA. 2020;**323**(18):1824-1836. DOI: 10.1001/jama.2020.6019

[16] Hossen MS, Barek MA, Jahan N, Safiqul Islam M. A review on current repurposing drugs for the treatment of COVID-19: Reality and challenges. SN Comprehensive Clinical Medicine.

2020;**2**(10):1777-1789. DOI: 10.1007/s42399-020-00485-9

[17] Collaborative Recovery Group. Tocilizumab in patients admitted to the hospital with COVID-19 (RECOVERY): A randomized, controlled, open, platform trial. Lancet. 2021;**397**(10285):1637-1645

[18] Tomazini BM, Maia IS, Bueno FR, et al. COVID-19-associated ARDS treated with DEXamethasone (CoDEX): Study design and rationale for a randomized trial. Revista Brasileira de Terapia Intensiva, [S.L.] (GN1 Genesis Network). 2020;**32**(3):354-362. DOI: 10.5935/0103-507x.20200063. Disponível em: https://www.scielo.br/j/rbti/a/b7fXwJt3KTmc4zhM7p8vKhf/?lang=en. Acesso em: 21 abr. 2021

[19] Schakman O, Kalista S, Barbé C, et al. Glucocorticoid-induced skeletal muscle atrophy. The International Journal of Biochemistry & Cell Biology, [S.L.] (Elsevier BV). out. 2013;**45**(10):2163-2172. DOI: 10.1016/j.biocel.2013.05.036. Disponível em: https://www.sciencedirect.com/science/article/abs/pii/S1357272513001817?via%3Dihub. Acesso em: 07 fev. 2021

[20] Hermans G, Berghe GVD. Clinical review: Intensive care unit acquired weakness. Critical Care, [S.L.] (Springer Science and Business Media LLC). dez 2015;**19**(1):1-9. DOI: 10.1186/s13054-015-0993-7. Disponível em: https://ccforum.biomedcentral.com/articles/10.1186/s13054-015-0993-7. Acesso em: 06 abr. 2021

[21] Park HY, Jung J, Park HY, Lee SH, Kim ES, Kim HB, et al. Psychological consequences of survivors of COVID-19 pneumonia 1 month after discharge. Journal of Korean Medical Science. 2020;**35**(47):e409. DOI: 10.3346/jkms.2020.35.e409

[22] Shang L, Zhao J, Hu Y, et al. On the use of corticosteroids for 2019-nCoV pneumonia. The Lancet, [S.L.] (Elsevier BV). fev 2020;**395**(10225):683-684. DOI: 10.1016/s0140-6736(20)30361-5. Disponível em: https://www.ncbi.nlm.nih.gov/pmc/articles/PMC7159292/. Acesso em: 10 fev. 2021

[23] Horby P, Lim WS, Emberson JR. Dexamethasone in hospitalized patients with Covid-19: Preliminary report. New England Journal of Medicine, [S.L.] (Massachusetts Medical Society). 25 fev. 2021;**384**(8):693-704. DOI: 10.1056/nejmoa2021436. Disponível em: https://www.nejm.org/doi/suppl/10.1056/NEJMoa2021436/suppl_file/nejmoa2021436_preliminary.pdf. Acesso em: 05 abr. 2021

[24] Rhen T, Cidlowski JA. Antiinflammatory action of glucocorticoids — New mechanisms for old drugs. New England Journal of Medicine, [S.L.] (Massachusetts Medical Society). 20 out. 2005;**353**(16):1711-1723. DOI: 10.1056/nejmra050541. Disponível em: https://www.nejm.org/doi/10.1056/NEJMra050541?url_ver=Z39.88-2003&rfr_id=ori%3Arid%3Acrossref.org&rfr_dat=cr_pub++0pubmed. Acesso em: 09 fev. 2021

[25] Meduri GU, Siemieniuk RAC, et al. Prolonged low-dose methylprednisolone treatment is highly effective in reducing duration of mechanical ventilation and mortality in patients with ARDS. Journal of Intensive Care, [S.L.] (Springer Science and Business Media LLC). 24 ago. 2018;**6**(1):1-7. DOI: 10.1186/s40560-018-0321-9. Disponível em: https://jintensivecare.biomedcentral.com/articles/10.1186/s40560-018-0321-9#citeas. Acesso em: 09 fev. 2021

[26] Ko JJ, Wu C, Mehta N, et al. A comparison of methylprednisolone and dexamethasone in intensive care patients

with COVID-19. Journal of Intensive Care Medicine, [S.L.] (SAGE Publications). 25 fev. 2021;**36**(6):673-680. DOI: 10.1177/0885066621994057. Disponível em: https://journals.sagepub.com/doi/10.1177/0885066621994057?url_ver=Z39.88-2003&rfr_id=ori%3Arid%3Acrossref.org&rfr_dat=cr_pub++0pubmed&. Acesso em: 06 jul. 2021

[27] Paddon-Jones D, Sheffield-Moore M, Cree MG, et al. Atrophy and impaired muscle protein synthesis during prolonged inactivity and stress. The Journal of Clinical Endocrinology & Metabolism, [S.L.] (The Endocrine Society). 1 dez. 2006;**91**(12):4836-4841. DOI: 10.1210/jc.2006-0651. Disponível em: https://academic.oup.com/jcem/article/91/12/4836/2656308. Acesso em: 10 maio 2021

[28] Mayer KP, Bastin MLT, Montgomery-Yates AA. et al. Acute skeletal muscle wear and dysfunction predict physical disability at hospital discharge in patients with critical illness. Critical Care. 2021;**24**(1)

[29] Kirwan R, McCullough D, Butler T, Perez de Heredia F, Davies IG, Stewart C. Sarcopenia during COVID-19 lockdown restrictions: Long-term health effects of short-term muscle loss. GeroScience. 2020;**42**(6):1547-1578. DOI: 10.1007/s11357-020-00272-3

[30] Villar J, Ferrando C, Martínez D, et al. Dexamethasone treatment for the acute respiratory distress syndrome: A multicentre, randomised controlled trial. The Lancet Respiratory Medicine, [S.L.] (Elsevier BV). mar. 2020;**8**(3):267-276. DOI: 10.1016/s2213-2600(19)30417-5. Disponível em: https://www.thelancet.com/journals/lanres/article/PIIS2213-2600(19)30417-5/fulltext. Acesso em: 05 mar. 2021

[31] Lheureux O, Prevedello D, Preiser JC. Update on glucose in critical care. Nutrition, [S.L.] (Elsevier BV). mar. 2019;**59**:14-20. DOI: 10.1016/j.nut.2018.06.027. Disponível em: https://pubmed.ncbi.nlm.nih.gov/30415158/. Acesso em: 09 maio 2021

[32] Veiga VC, Prats JA, Farias DL, et al. Effect of tocilizumab on clinical outcomes at 15 days in patients with severe or critical coronavirus disease 2019: Randomized controlled trial. The BMJ. 2021;**2021**:372

[33] REACT Rapid Evidence Appraisal for COVID-19 Therapies (REACT) Working Group. Association between administration of IL-6 antagonists and mortality among patients hospitalized for COVID-19. Jama, [S.L.] (American Medical Association (AMA)). 10 ago. 2021;**326**(6):499-518. DOI: 10.1001/jama.2021.11330. Disponível em: https://jamanetwork.com/journals/jama/fullarticle/2781880#full-text-tab. Acesso em: 10 set. 2021

[34] Tournadre A, Pereira B, Dutheil F, Giraud C, Courteix D, Sapin V, et al. Changes in body composition and metabolic profile during interleukin 6 inhibition in rheumatoid arthritis. Journal of Cachexia, Sarcopenia and Muscle. 2017;**8**(4):639-646. DOI: 10.1002/jcsm.12189

[35] Tleyjeh IM, Kashour Z, Riaz M, et al. Efficacy and safety of tocilizumab in COVID-19 patients: A living systematic review and meta-analysis, first update. Clinical Microbiology And Infection, [S.L.] (Elsevier BV). ago. 2021;**27**(8):1076-1082. DOI: 10.1016/j.cmi.2021.04.019. Disponível em: https://www.clinicalmicrobiologyandinfection.com/article/S1198-743X(21)00204-4/fulltext. Acesso em: 07 maio 2021

[36] Ghosn L, Chaimani A, Evrenoglou T, et al. Interleukin-6 blocking agents for treating COVID-19: A living systematic

review. Cochrane Database of Systematic Reviews, [S.L.] (Wiley). 18 mar. 2021;**2021**(3). DOI: 10.1002/14651858.cd013881. Disponível em: https://www.cochranelibrary.com/cdsr/doi/10.1002/14651858.CD013881/full/pt#CD013881-abs-0005. Acesso em: 06 jul. 2021

[37] REMAP-CAP Investigators, Gordon AC, Mouncey PR, Al-Beidh F, Rowan KM, Nichol AD, et al. Interleukin-6 receptor antagonists in critically Ill patients with Covid-19. The New England Journal of Medicine. 2021;**384**(16):1491-1502. DOI: 10.1056/NEJMoa2100433

[38] Roche. Results of the Ab Cocktail Report (Casirivimab + Imdevimab) in P-III REGN-COV 2069 Covid Symptomatic Infection Assay 19. 2021. Available from: https://pharmashots.com/58368/roche-report-results-of-ab-cocktail-casirivimab-imdevimab-in-p-iii-regncov-2069-trial-for-symptomatic-covid-19-infection/

[39] Weinreich DM, Sivapalasingam S, Norton T. REGN-COV2, a neutralizing antibody cocktail, in outpatients with Covid-19. New England Journal of Medicine. 2021;**384**(3):238-251

[40] Klok F, Kruip MJ, Van Meer NJ, Arbous MS, Gommers DA, et al. Incidence of thrombotic complications in ICU patients who are seriously ill with COVID-19. Thrombotic Research. 2020;**10**:301

[41] Shi C, Wang C, Wang H, Yang C, Cai F, Zeng F et al. The potential for low molecular weight heparin to mitigate cytokine storm in severe COVID-19 patients: A retrospective clinical study. medRxiv. 2020;**13**(6):1087-1095

[42] Langford BJ, So M, Raybardhan S, Leung V, Westwood D, Macfadden DR, et al. Bacterial co-infection and secondary infection in patients with COVID-19: Rapid review and live meta-analysis. Clinical microbiology and infection: Official publication of the European Society of Clinical Microbiology and Infectious Diseases. 2020;**26**(12):1622-1629. DOI: 10.1016/j.cmi.2020.07.016

[43] Ranzani OT, Bastos LL, Gelli JGM, et al. Characterisation of the first 250 000 hospital admissions for COVID-19 in Brazil: A retrospective analysis of nationwide data. The Lancet Respiratory Medicine, [S.L.] (Elsevier BV). abr. 2021;**9**(4):407-418. DOI: 10.1016/s2213-2600(20)30560-9. Disponível em: https://www.arca.fiocruz.br/handle/icict/46140. Acesso em: 07 abr. 2021

[44] World Health Organization. Corticosteroids for COVID-19. Living Guidance. 2020. Retrieved from https://www.who.int/publications/i/item/WHO-2019-nCoV-Corticosteroids-2020.1

[45] Alhazzani W, Evans L, Alshamsi F, et al. Surviving sepsis campaign guidelines on the management of adults with coronavirus disease 2019 (COVID-19) in the ICU: First update. Critical Care Medicine, [S.L.] (Ovid Technologies (Wolters Kluwer Health)). 28 jan. 2021;**49**(3):219-234. DOI: 10.1097/ccm.0000000000004899. Disponível em: https://journals.lww.com/ccmjournal/Fulltext/2021/03000/Surviving_Sepsis_Campaign_Guidelines_on_the.21.aspx. Acesso em: 05 mar. 2021

[46] Kernick J, Magarey J. What is the evidence for the use of high flow nasal cannula oxygen in adult patients admitted to critical care units? A systematic review. Australian Critical Care, [S.L.] (Elsevier BV). maio 2010;**23**(2):53-70. DOI: 10.1016/j.aucc.2010.01.001. Disponível em: https://www.australiancriticalcare.com/article/S1036-7314(10)00002-0/fulltext. Acesso em: 10 maio 2021

[47] Yuste ME, Moreno O, Narbona S, et al. Efficacy and safety of high-flow nasal cannula oxygen therapy in moderate acute hypercapnic respiratory failure. Revista Brasileira de Terapia Intensiva, [S.L.] (GN1 Genesis Network). 2019;**31**(2):156-163. DOI: 10.5935/0103-507x.20190026. Disponível em: https://www.scielo.br/j/rbti/a/QNGPTVv7w4MwLPhQ8wt97fK/?lang=pt. Acesso em: 10 maio 2021

[48] Dysart K, Miller TL, Wolfson MR, et al. Research in high flow therapy: Mechanisms of action. Respiratory Medicine, [S.L.] (Elsevier BV). out. 2009;**103**(10):1400-1405. DOI: 10.1016/j.rmed.2009.04.007. Disponível em: https://www.resmedjournal.com/article/S0954-6111(09)00132-2/fulltext. Acesso em: 05 maio 2021

[49] Sotello D, Rivas M, Mulkey Z, et al. High-Flow nasal cannula oxygen in adult patients: A narrative review. The American Journal of the Medical Sciences, [S.L.] (Elsevier BV). fev. 2015;**349**(2):179-185. DOI: 10.1097/maj.0000000000000345. Disponível em: https://www.amjmedsci.org/article/S0002-9629(15)30126-9/fulltext. Acesso em: 05 maio 2021

[50] Cai H, Chen Y, Chen Z, et al. Handbook of COVID-19 Prevention an Treatment. The first Affiliated Hospital, Zhejiang University School of Medicine, 2020. Australian and New Zealand Intensive Care Society. ANZICS COVID-19 Guidelines, 2020. Melbourne: ANZICS; 2020

[51] Cordeiro ALL. Manual de Ventilação Mecânica nas Afecções Virais. Salvador: Sanar; 2020. p. 352

[52] Piraino T. Noninvasive respiratory support in acute hypoxemic respiratory failure. Respiratory Care, [S.L.] (Daedalus Enterprises). 20 maio 2019;**64**(6):638-646. DOI: 10.4187/respcare.06735. Disponível em: http://rc.rcjournal.com/content/64/6/638/tab-pdf. Acesso em: 09 maio 2021

[53] Whittle JS, Pavlov I, Sacchetti AD, et al. Respiratory support for adult patients with COVID-19. Journal of the American College of Emergency Physicians Open, [S.L.] (Wiley). abr. 2020;**1**(2):95-101. DOI: 10.1002/emp2.12071. Disponível em: https://www.ncbi.nlm.nih.gov/pmc/articles/PMC7228246/. Acesso em: 10 maio 2021

[54] Spadari JAA, Gardenghi G. Aspectos fisiopatológicos do COVID-19 e uso de ventilação não invasiva. É possível? Revista Pesquisa em Fisioterapia, [S.L.] (Escola Bahiana de Medicina e Saude Publica). 4 ago. 2020;**10**(3):372-375. DOI: 10.17267/2238-2704rpf.v10i3.3036. Disponível em: https://www5.bahiana.edu.br/index.php/fisioterapia/article/view/3036. Acesso em: 09 maio 2021

[55] Ranieri VM, Rubenfeld GD, Thompson BT. The ARDS definition task force. Acute respiratory distress syndrome. Jama, [S.L.] (American Medical Association (AMA)). 20 jun. 2012;**307**(23):2526-2533. DOI: 10.1001/jama.2012.5669

[56] Gattinoni L, Chiumello D, Rossi S. COVID-19 pneumonia: Ards or not? Critical Care, [S.L.] (Springer Science and Business Media LLC). 16 abr. 2020;**24**(1):1-3. DOI: 10.1186/s13054-020-02880-z. Disponível em: https://ccforum.biomedcentral.com/articles/10.1186/s13054-020-02880-z#citeas. Acesso em: 10 maio 2021

[57] Sarmento GJV. Fisioterapia respiratória de A a Z. Barueri: Manole; 2016

[58] Inoue S, Hatakeyama J, Kondo Y, et al. Post-intensive care syndrome: Its pathophysiology, prevention, and future

directions. Acute Medicine & Surgery, [S.L.] (Wiley). 25 abr. 2019;**6**(3):233-246. DOI: 10.1002/ams2.415. Acesso em: 10 maio 2021

[59] Jones C, Eddleston J, Mccairn A, et al. Improving rehabilitation after critical illness through outpatient physiotherapy classes and essential amino acid supplement: A randomized controlled trial. Journal of Critical Care, [S.L.] (Elsevier BV). out. 2015;**30**(5):901-907. DOI: 10.1016/j.jcrc.2015.05.002. Acesso em: 06 jun. 2021

[60] Bonorino KC, Cani KC. Early mobilization in the time of COVID-19. Revista Brasileira de Terapia Intensiva, [S.L.] (GN1 Genesis Network). 2020;**32**(4):484-486. DOI: 10.5935/0103-507x.20200086. Disponível em: http://rbti.org.br/artigo/detalhes/0103507X-32-4-1. Acesso em: 11 out. 2021

[61] Puthucheary ZA, Rawal J, McPhail M, Connolly B, Ratnayake G, Chan P, et al. Acute skeletal muscle wasting in critical illness. JAMA. 2013;**310**(15):1591-1600. DOI: 10.1001/jama.2013.278481

[62] Costa-Beber LC, Hirsch GE, Heck TG, et al. Companion duality: The role of extracellular and intracellular hsp70 as a biomarker of endothelial dysfunction in the development of atherosclerosis. Archives of Physiology and Biochemistry. 2020;**2020**:1-8

[63] Fraser DD, Cepinskas G, Slessarev M, et al. Inflammation profile of patients with severely ill coronavirus disease 2019. Care Exploration Reviews. 2020;**2**(6):144

[64] Gabay C, Kushner I. Acute phase proteins and other systemic responses to inflammation. New England Journal of Medicine. 1999;**340**(6):448

[65] Guo SC, Xu CW, Liu YQ, et al. Changes in plasmalevels of thrombomodulin and D-dimer in children with different types of mycoplasma pneumoniae pneumonia. Zhongguo Dang Dai Er Ke Za Zhi. 2013;**15**(8):619

[66] Halpern NO, Pastores SM. Critical medicine in the United States 2000-2005: An analysis of bed numbers, occupancy rates, mix of payers and costs. Critical Care Medicine. 2021;**38**(1):65

[67] Heck TG, Ludwig ES, Frizzo MN, et al. Suppressed anti-inflammatory thermal shock response in high-risk covid-19 patients: Basic research lessons (inclusive bats), light on conceivable therapies. Clinical Science. 2020;**134**(15):1991

[68] Herold T, Jurinovic V, Arnreich C, et al. High levels of IL-6 and CRP predict the need for mechanical ventilation in COVID-19. Journal of Allergy and Clinical Immunology. 2020;**146**(1):128

[69] Hui P, Cook DJ, Lim W, et al. The frequency and clinical significance of thrombocytopenia complicating critical disease. Breast. 2011;**139**(2):271

[70] Jager CPC, Wever PC, Gemen EFA, et al. The neutron-lymphocyte count ratio in patients with community-acquired pneumonia. Plos One. 2012;**7**(10):46561

[71] Jin YH, Cai L, Cheng ZS, et al. A quick guidance of counseling for the diagnosis and treatment of the new coronavirus 2019 (2019-nCoV) infected pneumonia (standard version). Military Medical Research. 2021;**7**(1):1

[72] Letko M, Marzi A, Munster V. Functional evaluation of cell input and receptor use for SARS-CoV-2 and other betacoronavirus B salling. Nature Microbiology. 2021;**5**(4):562-569

[73] Lippi G, Plebani M, Henry BM. Thrombocytopenia is associated

with severe coronavirus disease infections 2019 (COVID-19): A meta-analysis. Clinica Chimica Acta. 2020;**506**:145-148

[74] Liu F, Li L, Xu M, et al. Prognostic value of interleukin-6, C-reactive protein and procalcitonin in patients with COVID-19. Journal of Clinical Virology. 2020;**127**:104370

[75] Liu J, Liu Y, Xiang P, et al. The neutrophil-lymphocyte relationship predicts patients with critical disease with early-stage coronavirus disease 2019. Journal of Translational Medicine. 2021;**18**:1

[76] Long L, Zeng X, Zhang X, et al. Short-term outcomes of COVID-19 and risk factors for progression. European Respiratory Journal. 2021;**55**:200

[77] Macario AJ, Macario EC. Molecular mechanisms in chapeopathies: Clues to understand histopathological abnormalities and develop new therapies. The Journal of Pathology. 2019;**250**:9

[78] Mitaka C. Clinical laboratory differentiation of infectious versus non-infectious systemic inflammatory response syndrome. Clinica Chimica Acta. 2005;**351**:17

[79] Moore JB, June HC. Cytokine release syndrome in severe COVID-19. Science. 2020;**368**:6490

[80] Paladino L, Vitale AM, Bavisotto DC, et al. The role of molecular companions in virus infection and implications for the understanding and treatment of COVID-19. Journal of Clinical Medicine. 2020;**9**:3518

[81] Qu R, Ling Y, Zhang YH, Wei LY, et al. Platelet--para-lymphocyte ratio is associated with prognosis in patients with coronavirus disease-19. Journal of Medical Virology. 2020;**92**:1533

[82] Gordon AC, Mouncey PR, Al-Beidh F, Rowan KM, Nichol AD, Arabi YM, et al. Interleukin-6 receptor antagonists in critically ill patients with Covid-19 - Preliminary report. medRxiv. 2021;**384**(16):1491-1502

[83] Ruan Q, Yang K, Wang W, et al. Clinical predictors of mortality due to COVID-19 based on a data analysis of 150 patients from Wuhan, China. Intensive Care Medicine. 2021;**46**:846

[84] Tan C, Huang Y, Shi F, et al. C-reactive protein correlates with computed tomographic findings and predicts severe covid-19 early. Journal of Medical Virology. 2021a;**92**:856

[85] Tan L, Wang Q, Zhang D, Ding J, Huang Q, et al. The lymphogin predicts the severity of COVID-19 disease: A descriptive and predictive study. Signal Transduction and Directed Therapy. 2021b;**5**:33

[86] Ye W, Chen G, Li X, et al. Dynamic changes in d-dimer and neutrophil-lymphocyte counts as prognostic biomarkers in COVID-19. Respiratory Research. 2021;**21**:169

[87] Zhang M, Tan J, Xu Y, Song R. The neutrophil-lymphocyte relationship predicts patients with critical disease with early-stage coronavirus disease 2019. Journal of Translational Medicine. 2020;**18**:12

Chapter 8

COVID-19 Drug Development: Role of Drug Repurposing

Kenneth Bitrus David, Yusuff Azeez Olanrewaju and Cynthia Chidera Okafor

Abstract

The COVID-19 pandemic came at a time when the scientific world was least prepared for it. It emerged at a time when there were variable research availability and limited mechanistic insights about the virus. Amid these challenges, research works were carried out in a bid to discover ways of curbing the spread of the virus and improving the health outcome of the population. Drug repurposing was one concept that was explored by scientists. Through this concept, already existing drugs were repurposed for the treatment of COVID-19, with incredible results seen. This chapter provides insights on some repurposed drugs, steps taken in drug repurposing, challenges peculiar to the methods, and a framework for continuity.

Keywords: drug repurposing, COVID-19, drug development, pandemic

1. Introduction

Coronaviruses, a large group of positive-sense RNA, single-stranded, and enveloped viruses have been one of the viral sources of respiratory diseases [1]. In December 2019, they caught the attention of the world when a strain of the virus-n-CoV-19, which was later renamed SARS-CoV-2 virus-caused epidemic cases of respiratory tract infection in Wuhan, China. The initial cases were presumed to be complications of pneumonia and were treated as such, until when further studies were conducted as regards the rate of spread, morbidity, and mortality of the disease [2]. Findings from studies conducted provided evidence that made the World Health Organization (WHO) declare the disease as a global health emergency and subsequently a pandemic.

For the first 12 months since the inception of the pandemic, COVID-19 spread worldwide, gravely affecting countries such as Turkey, Iran, Poland, Mexico, Germany, Colombia, Argentina, Spain, Italy, United Kingdom, France, Russian Federation, Brazil, India, and the USA, with each country recording over 1 million confirmed cases (https://covid19.who.int/accessed on August 25, 2022). The lack of proper treatment and vaccine made the mortality rate quite high [3].

Some of the measures used in curbing the spread of the virus and improving the quality of life of those infected included national and international lockdown, travel restrictions, mandatory use of face covering, washing of hands, and social

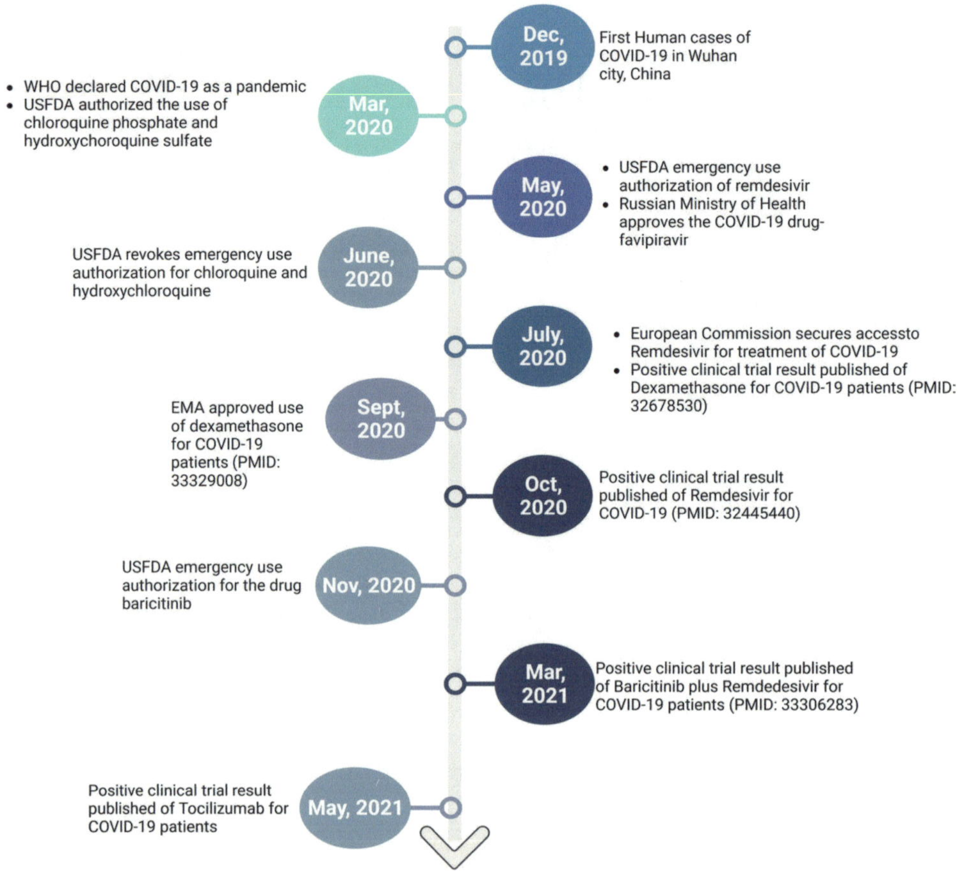

Figure 1.
Showing the timeline of the COVID-19 pandemic and details of repurposed drugs used [5–9].

distancing [4]. Also, some drugs were repurposed for the management of the disease, and vaccines were developed. **Figure 1** shows the timeline of the COVID-19 pandemic and details of some repurposed drugs used [5].

2. Historical overview of drug repurposing

Drug repurposing, also known as indication shift, indication expansion, drug proofing, or drug repositioning, involves establishing a new medical use for an already known drug. These drugs can be experimental, shelved, discontinued, or already approved. Although drug repurposing is not a new strategy, it has gained wide recognition in recent times in the pharmaceutical sector [10].

The procedure to authorize a new medicine is costly and can take 10–15 years. This drawn-out discovery process makes drug repurposing (repositioning) a viable alternative strategy for reducing the amount of time needed to produce medicine. This original concept of drug repositioning has since been expanded to encompass active ingredients that failed the clinical stage of their development due to their toxicity or insufficient efficacy, as well as medications pulled off the market due to safety concerns. However, compounds that have not yet been the focus of clinical research should not be included. This specifically disallows chemicals maintained in chemical libraries by academic and industrial research groups from being screened to find new biological qualities, apart from the properties for which they were initially developed and synthesized. Thus, any changes to the drug's structural makeup are not included in the idea of drug repositioning. Instead, repositioning uses either the biological properties for which the drug has already received approval (possibly in accordance with a different formulation, at a new dose, or via a new route of administration) or the side properties of a drug that are accountable for its negative effects in a new indication. The fact that various diseases share occasionally similar biological targets, as revealed by the elucidation of the human genome, and the idea of pleiotropic medications, serve as the two fundamental scientific foundations for therapeutic repositioning [11, 12]. Repurposing a medicine involves using it for a different indication after having it licensed by a regulatory body like the FDA, the European Medicines Agency (EMA), or the Medicines and Healthcare Products Regulatory Agency (MHRA), among others. Many pharmaceutical companies are presently using drug repurposing to regenerate some of their FDA-approved and previously unsuccessful pipeline molecules as novel medicines for a variety of illness conditions due to the enormous promise of a reduced development cycle [13, 14].

One of the keys to drug repurposing is the description of the factors related to the complicated interplay between diseases, medications, and targets using in silico methodologies (data mining, machine learning, ligand-based, and structure-based approaches). Today, diseases can be described in terms of their molecular profile (including the genes, biomarkers, signaling pathways, and environmental factors), and the degree of similarity between diseases that share a number of these molecular features can be assessed using computational methods, particularly data mining. Protein targets that are shared by a number of diseases imply that a given medication may be effective in treating both disorders [12, 15–17]. In terms of their core therapeutic effects and their (generally undesirable) side effects, the majority of medications are now phenotypically well described. The drug's pleiotropic interactions with a number of (primary and secondary) biological targets cause this variety of side effects. Therefore, if one of a medicine's secondary targets plays a part in an illness different than the one for which it was initially intended, the treatment may be effective against the new disease. Be aware that these pleiotropic interactions allow for the development of medications with many, intended effects that work in concert to increase clinical efficacy, such as the pan-kinase inhibitors used in cancer. Regardless of their therapeutic reason, medications can be analyzed for phenotypic similarities much like diseases are. A medicine may be successful for both indications if it has a high similarity score to another treatment designated for a separate condition [10, 16].

2.1 Significance of drug repurposing

Drug repurposing reduces the development cost for drugs because they have already gone through clinical trials, toxicity studies, and other tests [18]. **Tables 1** and **2** below show a list of some repurposed drugs in the past.A recent analysis based on a survey of 30 pharmaceutical and biotechnology companies found that the average cost to relaunch a repurposed drug is $8.4 million, compared to an average cost of $41.3 million for a new formulation of an existing drug in its original indication [20]. They have a higher success rate than the original drugs, owing to the availability of comprehensive information on their pharmacology, formulation, potential toxicity, safety, and adverse drug reaction issues, thereby reducing their attrition rate [21]. Since repurposing is based

S/N	Drug name	Original indication	New indication	Mechanism of action	Status of study	Ref.
1	Itraconazole	Antifungal	Prostate cancer	Reducing prostate-specific antigen (PSA) levels	Phase 2	[19]
2	Metformin	Type 2 Diabetes	Advanced prostate cancer	Inhibition of the mammalian target of rapamycin complex 1 (mTORC1) pathway	Phase 2	[19]
3	Aspirin	Fever and pain	Melanoma	Stop the growth of tumor cells by blocking some of the enzymes needed for cell growth	Phase 2	[11]
4	Sildenafil	Angina pectoris	Erectile dysfunction	Phosphodiesterase type 5 (PDE5) inhibition	Approved	[11]
5	Thalidomide	Morning sickness	Multiple myeloma	Antiangiogenic	Approved	[11]
6	Sodium Nitrite	Antidote to cyanide poisoning	Chronic leg ulcers associated with sickle cell and other blood disorders	Vasodilation	Recruiting participants for clinical trial	[11]
7	Celebrex	Osteoarthritis	Reduce the risk of additional polyp formation in colon cancer	Inhibiting COX-2 receptors	Approved	[11]
8	Dapsone	Leprosy	Malaria	Inhibit bacterial dihydropteroate synthase	Phase 3 completed	[11]
9	Amphotericin	Antifungal	Leishmaniasis	Disruption of parasite membrane	Phase 3 completed	[11]
10	Eflornithine	Cancer	African trypanosomiasis	Inhibition of ornithine decarboxylase (ODC)	Phase 3 completed	[11]

Table 1.
List of some drugs that have been repurposed.

on prior research and development efforts, new drug candidates could be promptly prepared for clinical trials, hastening the FDA's review of them and, if approved, their introduction into healthcare, shortening the time it takes for the full processing cycle. Re-profiled medications also save the upfront costs and delays associated with bringing a drug to market, because it takes a great deal of time, money, and effort to produce a new medicine. In general, it frequently takes more than 15 years to convert a potential therapeutic candidate into an approved medication [22]. Therefore, it is essential to develop drug repurposing procedures in order to reduce the time and cost of drugs

S/No	Repurposed drug for COVID-19	Previous indication
1	Azithromycin	An antibiotic used for the treatment of respiratory and urinary tract infections
2	Mavrilimumab	Rheumatoid arthritis
3	Baricitinib	Rheumatoid arthritis
4	Hydroxychloroquine sulfate and chloroquine phosphate	Amoebic dysentery and malaria
5	Lopinavir-ritonavir	HIV/AIDS treatment and prevention
6	Favipiravir	Influenza
7	Dexamethasone	Asthma, allergies, skin diseases

Table 2.
List of some repurposed drugs for the treatment of COVID-19.

while also raising their success rates. In addition, repurposed compounds have a market penetration rate of 25% from Phase II and 65% from Phase III clinical trials, compared to 10% and 50%, respectively, for novel molecular entities [23].

For a new investigational molecule, safety and efficacy data are not yet available, resulting in higher attrition during the drug discovery process leading to the most failures regarding safety or efficacy. By contrast, all safety, preclinical, and efficacy data are readily available for a repurposed molecule, thus enabling the investigator to make an informed decision at each stage of drug development [23, 24]. Availability of prior knowledge regarding safety, efficacy, and the appropriate administration route significantly reduces the development costs and cuts down the development time resulting in less effort required for successfully bringing a repositioned drug to market [25]. For example, sildenafil, a phosphodiesterase type 5 (PDE5) inhibitor, represents one of the successful repurposing efforts. Sildenafil was originally developed for hypertension treatment but was later identified to have significant benefits in erectile dysfunction and was approved by the FDA for the same. It was later repurposed for the treatment of a rare disorder: pulmonary hypertension [26]. Also, daptomycin (an antibacterial agent) was repurposed for the treatment of Zika virus infection, chlorcyclizine (an antihistamine) was repurposed for the management of hepatitis C virus infection, and manidipine (an antihypertensive agent) was repurposed for Japanese encephalitis virus treatment [27].

3. Repurposed drugs for COVID-19 pandemic

Due to the urgent need for COVID-19 treatment options, all repurposed drugs were given emergency approval. Approval for hydroxychloroquine and chloroquine were later revoked due to the high number of cardiac toxicity recorded (**Figure 2**) [10].

4. A simplified scheme of the life cycle of SARS-CoV-2

Based on the likely mechanism by which registered pharmaceuticals combat the Coronavirus, the disease, or its symptoms, drug repurposing possibilities for COVID-19 can be categorized.

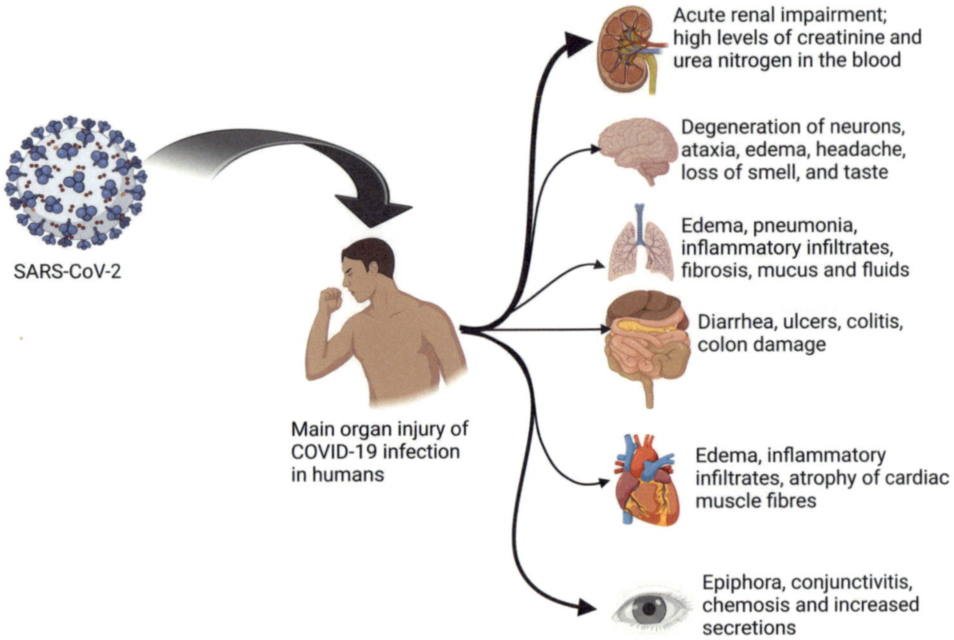

Figure 2.
Main organ injury of SARS-CoV-2 infection [24].

a. Drugs that disrupt the Coronavirus replication cycle.

b. Drugs that indirectly ameliorate the effects/symptoms of COVID-19 disease through direct influence on cellular immunity and metabolism.

4.1 Drugs that disrupt the Coronavirus replication cycle

The mechanism of many antiviral medications is hinged on the interruption of one or more replication phases of the virus.

4.1.1 Attachment and entry of the virus into the host cell

The first phase of the virus replication cycle is the attachment and entry of the virus into the host cell. There are two ways through which SARS-CoV-2 can gain entry into host cells. The first is through the binding interaction of SARS-COV-2 spike protein (S) with the ACE2 receptor and transmembrane protease serine 2 of the target cell (TMPRSS2), while the second is through endocytosis [28]. ACE2 is the coupling site for SARS-CoV-2 spike protein, while TMPRSS2 facilitates host cell entrance; therefore, some drugs that interfere with ACE2 or TMPRSS2 have the potential for being repurposed in the management of COVID-19 because they will prevent the entry of SARS-CoV-2 into host cells. In theory, drugs such as dexamethasone, estradiol, isotretinoin, retinoic acid, and spironolactone can influence the expression of ACE2, while drugs such as bicalutamide, bromhexine, camostat mesylate, and nafamostat act similarly with TMPRSS2 [28]. In an experiment involving SARS-CoV-2 spike pseudotyped virus, dexamethasone was found to bind to ACE2, preventing binding of the spike protein of the virus to ACE2 and preventing entry of the virus into the target cell [29]. This is the likely mechanism by which dexamethasone would find activity against SARS-CoV-2 as a repurposed drug. Similarly, bromhexine is a TMPRSS2 protease blocker that prevents viropexis of SARS-CoV-2 into target cells through its blocking effect on TMPRSS2 [28].

Viral attachment and entry into the host cell involve the attachment of spike protein of the SARS-CoV-2 to ACE2 and further involvement of TMPRSS2. If potential drugs for repurposing in COVID-19 treatment leverage their possible effects on ACE2 and TMPRSS2, then drugs that could influence the viral strike protein are also theoretically useful enough to be repurposed in COVID-19 treatment. One such drug is bamlanivimab.

Bamlanivimab is a recombinant human IgG1κ monoclonal antibody with activity against the spike (S) surface protein of SARS-CoV-2 itself, not the ACE2 or TMPRSS2 of the host cell [28]. Umifenovir and nelfinavir are antiviral medications. Umifenovir was previously used in the prophylaxis and management of influenza, while nelfinavir is an antiretroviral medication used in HIV. Umifenovir inhibits spike protein trimerization, while nelfinavir inhibits membrane fusion. This implies that both drugs have the potential for repurposing in COVID-19 management [28].

Endocytosis is a process through which cells take in foreign material by enveloping it with their membrane [29]. Research has shown that SARS-CoV-2 is capable of entering host cells by means of endocytosis. Drugs that prevent the entry of SARS-CoV-2 by endocytosis into the host cell can be repurposed in COVID-19. Such drugs include chloroquine, hydroxychloroquine, artemisinin, amodiaquine, chlorpromazine, niclosamide, imatinib, artesunate, baricitinib, verapamil, and amiodarone [28]. Many of these drugs work by inhibiting membrane fusion between SARS-CoV-2 spike protein and the host cell membrane.

4.1.2 Chloroquine and hydroxychloroquine

Chloroquine belongs to the chemical class of antimalarial medications called 4-aminoquinolines [30, 31]. Hydroxychloroquine (HCQ) is a derivative of chloroquine obtained by β-hydroxylation of the N-ethyl substituent of chloroquine to give hydroxychloroquine, which has a hydroxyl group at the end of the side chain. Chloroquine was known to be an effective drug in the treatment of malaria due to its high activity against the asexual erythrocytic forms of the plasmodium. This high profile of effectiveness was however affected negatively due to the growing cases of plasmodial resistance to available antimalarial agents. Although chloroquine was initially developed to treat malaria, the focus has largely shifted to its antirheumatic and antiviral activity. Over the past 20 years, a great deal of research has gone into the investigation of the antiviral effects of chloroquine [32].

As an antimalarial agent, chloroquine/hydroxychloroquine enters the feeding vacuoles of the malaria parasite where it prevents the conversion of heme (a toxic product of the breakdown of hemoglobin) to hemozoin (which is not harmful to the parasite). Accumulation of heme leads to the death of the malaria parasite.

As a repurposed drug for COVID-19, in order to prevent the fusion of SARS-CoV-2 with the host cell membranes, chloroquine/hydroxychloroquine is thought to work by blocking endocytic proteins and elevating the pH of the endosomes [33]. The endocytic pathway interference, sialic acid receptor blockage, limitation of pH-mediated spike (S) protein cleavage at the angiotensin-converting enzyme 2 (ACE2) binding site, and cytokine storm prevention are all part of the mechanism of action of chloroquine/hydroxychloroquine [34]. The major drawbacks of the use of chloroquine or hydroxychloroquine in COVID-19 treatment are adverse effects such as retinopathy, prolonged QT interval on the ECG, and cardiotoxicity [35]. Hydroxychloroquine is preferred to chloroquine due to its increased hydrophilic nature and decreased toxicity. Hydroxychloroquine is also better tolerated than chloroquine [36].

In recent years, rheumatoid arthritis, lupus erythematosus, and amoebic hepatitis have all been managed with chloroquine and its hydroxyl derivative, hydroxychloroquine as anti-inflammatory agents. Chloroquine exhibits potent antiviral action against a variety of DNA and RNA viruses, including HIV-1, Influenza A, Influenza B, Coronavirus (SARS-CoV2), and many more. Recent reports and published research revealed that chloroquine and hydroxychloroquine were linked to slowed COVID-19 progression and shorter symptom duration. In June 2020, however, FDA revokes the emergency use authorization of the use of both chloroquine and hydroxychloroquine in the management of COVID-19, thus discouraging its use [32, 33].

4.1.3 Viral replication

After attachment and entry of the virus into the host cell, the SARS-CoV-2 life cycle then proceeds to the release of the viral RNA genome into the cytoplasm and translation of the replicase genes, which develop the replicase transcriptase complex (RTC) [28]. RNA replication is carried out by RNA-dependent RNA polymerase RdRp, which is incorporated within the RTC [28, 37]. Favipiravir, tenofovir, sofosbuvir, clevudine, and a number of other drugs have been suggested for COVID-19 repurposing due to their inhibitory effect on RdRp [28, 38]. Remdesivir (in its active form) is a nucleoside analog that inhibits the SARS-CoV-2 RdRp thereby preventing further replication of SARS-CoV-2 [39]. Other RNA replication inhibitors include ivermectin, mefloquine, doxycycline, emtricitabine, and tacrolimus.

After viral RNA replication, comes the translation of viral structural proteins. Atazanavir, saquinavir, lopinavir, and ritonavir were considered repurposing candidates for COVID-19 based on their activity as protease inhibitors (just as they are HIV protease inhibitors). This phase involves proteolytic processing of viral proteins, thus the use of protease inhibitors to interfere with and prevent the translation of proteins [28].

4.1.4 Viral assembly and release

This phase comprises of formation of mature virions and exocytosis. Progeny viruses are assembled in the endoplasmic reticulum-Golgi intermediate complex following the synthesis and processing of the viral structural proteins and are then transported in vesicles to be released by exocytosis. Candidates for repurposing include antiviral medications that target this phase of SARS-CoV-2 replication. Oseltamivir and daclatasvir are such medications [28]. Daclatasvir inhibits viral assembly while oseltamivir inhibits virus release. Oseltamivir interacts with exocytosis-related elements, preventing the viral escape from the cell [40]. Oseltamivir is effective for a number of avian influenza virus strains and functions as a neuraminidase inhibitor against the influenza virus [41].

4.2 Drugs that indirectly ameliorate the effects/symptoms of COVID-19 disease through direct influence on cellular immunity and metabolism

This group of drugs acts by completely different mechanisms as they do not share structural similarities. Some of them include dapaglifozin, leflunomide, plitidepsin, nitazoxanide. Nitazoxanide demonstrates broad-spectrum antiviral action against several viral diseases. Nitazoxanide showed good in-vitro activity against SARS-CoV-2 in cell culture experiments, showing potential for repurposing in COVID-19 [41]. Nitazoxanide has shown great promise in vitro, with a low IC50 against SARS-CoV-2. Nitazoxanide phosphorylates protein kinases activated by dsRNA to increase phosphorylated kinases activated by dsRNA to increase phosphorylated factor 2α. Factor 2α is an intracellular protein possessing antiviral activities [28]. Despite the potential effectiveness of these drugs, further in vivo and clinical testing are required.

5. Conclusion

The COVID-19 pandemic, though unprecedented, gave room for new insights and perspectives in different sectors of the world, including drug development. Drug repurpose came in handy in the fight against the pandemic by providing tentative treatment options for the prevention and treatment of the virus.

Conflict of interest

The authors declare no conflict of interest.

Author details

Kenneth Bitrus David[1,2*], Yusuff Azeez Olanrewaju[3,4,5]
and Cynthia Chidera Okafor[3,5,6]

1 Faculty of Pharmaceutical Sciences, Kaduna State University, Kaduna, Nigeria

2 Pharmafluence, Kaduna, Nigeria

3 University of Ibadan, Oyo, Nigeria

4 Institute of Medical Research and Training (IMRAT), University College Hospital, Ibadan, Nigeria

5 Pharmacists Council of Nigeria, Abuja, Nigeria

6 University College Hospital, Ibadan, Nigeria

*Address all correspondence to: kennethdavidb@gmail.com

References

[1] Fan Y, Zhao K, Shi Z-L, Zhou P. Bat coronaviruses in China. Viruses. 2019;**11**(3):210

[2] Wang C, Horby PW, Hayden FG, Gao GF. A novel coronavirus outbreak of global health concern. Lancet. 2020;**395**(10223):470-473

[3] Singhal T. A review of coronavirus disease-2019 (COVID-19). Indian Journal of Pediatrics. 2020;**87**(4):281-286. DOI: 10.1007/s12098-020-03263-6

[4] Ramphul K, Mejias SG. Coronavirus disease: A review of a new threat to public health. Cureus. 2020;**12**(3):e7276. DOI: 10.7759/cureus.7276

[5] Chakraborty C, Sharma AR, Bhattacharya M, Agoramoorthy G, Lee SS. The drug repurposing for COVID-19 clinical trials provide very effective therapeutic combinations: Lessons learned from major clinical studies. Frontiers in Pharmacology. 2021;**18**(12):704205. DOI: 10.3389/fphar.2021.704205

[6] Horby P, Lim WS, Emberson JR, et al. Dexamethasone in Hospitalized Patients with Covid-19. The New England Journal of Medicine. 2021;**384**(8):693-704. DOI: 10.1056/NEJMoa2021436

[7] Gozzo L, Longo L, Vitale DC, Drago F. Dexamethasone treatment for Covid-19, a curious precedent highlighting a regulatory gap. Frontiers in Pharmacology. 2020;**30**(11):621934. DOI: 10.3389/fphar.2020.621934

[8] Beigel JH, Tomashek KM, Dodd LE, et al. Remdesivir for the treatment of Covid-19 - Final report. The New England Journal of Medicine. 2020;**383**(19):1813-1826. DOI: 10.1056/NEJMoa2007764

[9] Kalil AC, Patterson TF, Mehta AK, et al. Baricitinib plus remdesivir for hospitalized adults with covid-19. The New England Journal of Medicine. 2021;**384**(9):795-807. DOI: 10.1056/NEJMoa2031994

[10] Naylor S, Kauppi DM, Schonfeld JP. Therapeutic drug repurposing, repositioning and rescue part II: Business review. Drug Discovery World. 2015;**16**(2):57-72

[11] Medina-Enríquez MM, Lopez-León S, Carlos-Escalante JA, Aponte-Torres Z, Cuapio A, Wegman-Ostrosky T. ACE2: The molecular doorway to SARS-CoV-2. Cell & Bioscience. 2020;**10**(1):148

[12] Ng YL, Salim CK, Chu JJH. Drug repurposing for COVID-19: Approaches, challenges and promising candidates. Pharmacology & Therapeutics. 2021;**228**:107930

[13] Zhang Y, Hu S, Wang J, Xue Z, Wang C, Wang N. Dexamethasone inhibits SARS-CoV-2 spike pseudotyped virus viropexis by binding to ACE2. Virology. 2021;**554**:83-88

[14] Mikhaylov EN, Lyubimtseva TA, Vakhrushev AD, Stepanov D, Lebedev DS, Vasilieva EY, et al. Bromhexine hydrochloride prophylaxis of COVID-19 for medical personnel: A randomized open-label study. Tharmalingam J, editor. Interdisciplinary Perspectives on Infectious Diseases. 2022;**2022**:1-7

[15] Immunology for Pharmacy. Elsevier; 2012. Available from: https://linkinghub.elsevier.com/retrieve/pii/C20090403040

[16] Lawrenson AS, Cooper DL, O'Neill PM, Berry NG. Study of the

antimalarial activity of 4-aminoquinoline compounds against chloroquine-sensitive and chloroquine-resistant parasite strains. Journal of Molecular Modeling. 2018;**24**(9):237

[17] Enna SJ, Bylund DB. Elsevier Science (Firm). XPharm: The Comprehensive Pharmacology Reference. Amsterdam; Boston: Elsevier; 2008. Available from: https://www.sciencedirect.com/science/referenceworks/9780080552323

[18] Low ZY, Farouk IA, Lal SK. Drug repositioning: New approaches and future prospects for life-debilitating diseases and the COVID-19 pandemic outbreak. Viruses. 2020;**12**(9):1058. DOI: 10.3390/v12091058

[19] Ward P, Small I, Smith J, Suter P, Dutkowski R. Oseltamivir (Tamiflu®) and its potential for use in the event of an influenza pandemic. The Journal of Antimicrobial Chemotherapy. 2005;**55**(suppl_1):i5-i21

[20] Paul D, Sanap G, Shenoy S, Kalyane D, Kalia K, Tekade RK. Artificial intelligence in drug discovery and development. Drug Discovery Today. 2021;**26**(1):80-93. DOI: 10.1016/j.drudis.2020.10.010

[21] Dodds M, Xiong Y, Mouksassi S, Kirkpatrick CM, Hui K, Doyle E, et al. Model-informed drug repurposing: A pharmacometric approach to novel pathogen preparedness, response and retrospection. British Journal of Clinical Pharmacology. 2021;**87**(9):3388-3397. DOI: 10.1111/bcp.14760

[22] Dalton K, Byrne S. Role of the pharmacist in reducing healthcare costs: Current insights. Integrated Pharmacy Research & Practice. 2017;**6**:37-46. DOI: 10.2147/IPRP.S108047

[23] Uzunova K, Filipova E, Pavlova V, Vekov T. Insights into antiviral mechanisms of remdesivir, lopinavir/ritonavir and chloroquine/hydroxychloroquine affecting the new SARS-CoV-2. Biomedicine & Pharmacotherapy. 2020;**131**:110668

[24] Oprea TI, Mestres J. Drug repurposing: Far beyond new targets for old drugs. The AAPS Journal. 2012;**14**(4):759-763

[25] Satarker S, Ahuja T, Banerjee M, Dogra S, Agarwal T, et al. Hydroxychloroquine in COVID-19: Potential mechanism of action against SARS-CoV-2. Current Pharmacological Reports. 2020;**6**(5):203-211

[26] White NJ, Watson JA, Hoglund RM, Chan XHS, Cheah PY, Tarning J. COVID-19 prevention and treatment: A critical analysis of chloroquine and hydroxychloroquine clinical pharmacology. PLoS Medicine. 2020;**17**(9):e1003252

[27] Mercorelli B, Palù G, Loregian A. Drug repurposing for viral infectious diseases: How far are we? Trends in Microbiology. 2018;**26**(10):865-876. DOI: 10.1016/j.tim.2018.04.004

[28] Parvathaneni V, Kulkarni NS, Muth A, Gupta V. Drug repurposing: A promising tool to accelerate the drug discovery process. Drug Discovery Today. 2019;**24**(10):2076-2085

[29] U.S. Food and Drug Administration. The Drug Development Process; 2022. Available from: https://www.fda.gov/patients/learn-about-drug-and-device-approvals/drug-development-process [Accessed 6 October 2022]

[30] Iwata H, Sawada R, Mizutani S, Yamanishi Y. Systematic drug repositioning for a wide range of diseases with integrative analyses of phenotypic and molecular data. Journal

of Chemical Information and Modeling. 2015;**55**(2):446-459

[31] March-Vila E, Pinzi L, Sturm N, Tinivella A, Engkvist O, Chen H, et al. On the integration of in silico drug design methods for drug repurposing. Frontiers in Pharmacology. 2017:8

[32] US FDA. FDA cautions against use of hydroxychloroquine or chloroquine for COVID-19 outside of the hospital setting or a clinical trial due to risk of heart rhythm problems. 2021. Available from: https://www.fda.gov/drugs/drug-safety-and-availability/fda-cautions-against-use-hydroxychloroquine-or-chloroquine-covid-19-outside-hospital-setting-or [Accessed: September 2, 2022]

[33] WHO. WHO discontinues hydroxychloroquine and lopinavir/ritonavir treatment arms for COVID-19. 2021. Available from: https://www.who.int/news/item/04-07-2020-who-discontinues-hydroxychloroquine-and-lopinavir-ritonavir-treatment-arms-for-covid-19#:~:text=WHO%20today%20accepted%20the%20re-commendation,19%20treatment%20for%20hospitalized%20patients. [Accessed: September 2, 2022]

[34] Arrowsmith J. Phase III and submission failures: 2007-2010. Nature Reviews. Drug Discovery. 2011;**10**(2):87-87

[35] Arrowsmith J. Phase II failures: 2008-2010. Nature Reviews. Drug Discovery. 2011;**10**(5):328-329

[36] Padhy B, Gupta Y. Drug repositioning: Re-investigating existing drugs for new therapeutic indications. Journal of Postgraduate Medicine. 2011;**57**(2):153

[37] Gatta G, van der Zwan JM, Casali PG, Siesling S, Dei Tos AP, Kunkler I, et al. Rare cancers are not so rare: The rare cancer burden in Europe. European Journal of Cancer. 2011;**47**(17):2493-2511

[38] Shineman DW, Alam J, Anderson M, Black SE, Carman AJ, Cummings JL, et al. Overcoming obstacles to repurposing for neurodegenerative disease. Annals of Clinical Translational Neurology. 2014;**1**(7):512-518

[39] Ashburn TT, Thor KB. Drug repositioning: Identifying and developing new uses for existing drugs. Nature Reviews. Drug Discovery. 2004;**3**(8):673-683

[40] Novac N. Challenges and opportunities of drug repositioning. Trends in Pharmacological Sciences. 2013;**34**(5):267-272

[41] Alghandour R, Ebrahim MA, Elshal AM, Ghobrial F, Elzaafarany M, ELbaiomy MA. Repurposing metformin as anticancer drug: Randomized controlled trial in advanced prostate cancer (MANSMED). Urologic Oncology. 2021;**39**(12):831.e1-831.e10. DOI: 10.1016/j.urolonc.2021.05.020